W0050505

TOPICS IN TOPICALS

TOPICS IN TOPICALS

Current Trends in the Formulation of
Topical Agents

Edited by
R. Marks
Department of Medicine
University of Wales College of Medicine
Cardiff

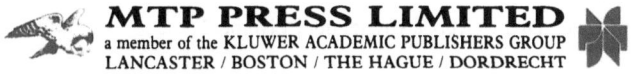
MTP PRESS LIMITED
a member of the KLUWER ACADEMIC PUBLISHERS GROUP
LANCASTER / BOSTON / THE HAGUE / DORDRECHT

Published in the UK and Europe by
MTP Press Limited
Falcon House
Lancaster, England

British Library Cataloguing in Publication Data

Topics in topicals: current trends in the
    formulation of topical agents.
    1. Skin—Diseases—Chemotherapy
    2. Dermatopharmacology
    I. Marks, R.
    615'.778   RL110

Published in the USA by
MTP Press
A division of Kluwer Boston Inc
190 Old Derby Street
Hingham, MA 02043, USA

Library of Congress Cataloging in Publication Data

Main entry under title:

Topics in topicals.

    Includes bibliographies and index.
    1. Dermatopharmacology.   2. Drugs—Dosage forms.
I. Marks, Ronald.
RL801.T67 1984   615'.778   84-23404
ISBN-13: 978-94-010-8673-8   e-ISBN-13: 978-94-009-4906-5
DOI: 10.1007/978-94-009-4906-5

Typesetting by Georgia Origination, Liverpool

Contents

List of Contributors

Dr M. I. Barnett
The Welsh School of Pharmacy
University of Wales Institute of
   Science and Technology
King Edward VII Avenue
Cardiff
CF1 3NU

Professor B. W. Barry
Postgraduate School of Studies in
   Pharmacy
University of Bradford
Bradford, W. Yorks
BD7 1DP

Dr A. Bashir
Department of Cardiology
University of Wales College of
   Medicine
Heath Park
Cardiff
CF4 4XN

Dr W. J. Cunliffe
The General Infirmary at Leeds
Great George Street
Leeds
LS1 3EX

Dr M. I. Foreman
Organon Laboratories Ltd
Newhouse
Lanarkshire
ML1 5SH

Dr J. Hadgraft
Department of Pharmacy
The University of Nottingham
University Park
Nottingham
NG7 2RD

Professor A. H. Henderson
Department of Cardiology
University of Wales College of
   Medicine
Heath Park
Cardiff
CF4 4XN

Professor I. W. Kellaway
The Welsh School of Pharmacy
University of Wales Institute of
   Science and Technology
King Edward VII Avenue
Cardiff
CF1 3NU

Dr M. J. Lewis
Departments of Pharmacology and
   Therapeutics
University of Wales College of
   Medicine
Heath Park,
Cardiff
CF4 4XN

Professor R. Marks
Department of Medicine
University of Wales College of
   Medicine
Heath Park
Cardiff
CF4 4XN

Dr J. R. Morgan
Department of Bacteriology
University of Wales College of
   Medicine
Heath Park
Cardiff
CF4 4XN

Dr R. C. Scott
Central Toxicology Laboratory
Imperial Chemical Industries PLC
Alderley Park
Nr. Macclesfield
Cheshire
SK10 4TJ

Introduction

Substances that are applied to the skin to heal it, make it feel better or improve its appearance, have much in common. They can all do damage to the skin as well as perform the task for which they were designed. They and the substances they contain are all absorbed through the skin to a greater or lesser extent. In addition, all these agents are constructed in the same general way. For these reasons it seems odd and uneconomical to consider topical pharmaceuticals, toiletry products and cosmetics separately. This was the reasoning behind the holding of a small symposium of workers involved with one or another aspect of the formulation of substances destined for application to the skin. Several aspects of the subject are covered in this book which is based on the symposium and the contents should be of interest to all who are concerned with the prescription, assessment or formulation of topical agents.

1
Acne Caused and Treated by Topical Agents

W. J. CUNLIFFE

The four main aetiological factors involved in the development of acne are (1) an elevated sebum excretion rate[1]; (2) ductal hyperkeratinization[2]; (3) an abnormality of microbial function[3]; (4) host inflammatory response[4]. Although opinions differ on both sides of the Atlantic, most authorities in the United Kingdom believe that increased sebum excretion rate is the main drive to acne, there being a definitive relationship between the severity of the acne and the seborrhoea of this disease.

The aim of this paper is to discuss factors which induce or treat acne by topical application.

TOPICAL INDUCTION OF ACNE

In this section the topical induction of acne by substances which affect sebum excretion, ductal microflora, mediators of inflammation and ductal hyperkeratinization will be considered.

Topical induction by altering sebum production

Androgens are the major causative factor in acne[5]. The topical application of androgens to one side of the forehead will increase the sebum excretion on that side. Androgens are absorbed and if applied in large enough amounts will increase sebum excretion at other sites. However, this effect is seen only in prepubertal subjects, and to some extent in adult females, and has virtually no effect in adult males since their sebaceous glands are maximally stimulated. Whether or not the topical application of androgens will actually precipitate acne has not been proven clinically, as topical therapy with androgens is not commonly used in the treatment of skin diseases. Nevertheless it is theoretically possible that the long-term application of topical androgens in prepubertal subjects and in females with a low sebum excretion would induce acne.

Topical induction by altering the microflora

Experimental evidence shows that polythene occlusion to the skin increases the number of the normal bacterial flora at that site, and a whole range of inflammatory lesions can be produced by polythene occlusion if a pathogenic strain is placed beneath it[6]. We know that acne may be induced under conditions of high humidity but there are no laboratory data to help us decide whether or not this induction is due to a change in the microflora. There is evidence to suggest that changes in the microenvironment, and consequently in the microflora, influence the development of acne vulgaris[7]. The topical application of corticosteroids will also induce acne. The mechanism, however, is uncertain. It may cause hyperkeratinization of the pilosebaceous duct[8]. Recent studies using betamethasone valerate as the corticosteroid of choice failed to demonstrate an increase in the number of *Propionibacterium acnes*, which is probably the most important organism involved in acne[9].

Topical induction by mediators of inflammation

It is unlikely that the acne vulgaris will be precipitated by the topical application of substances inducing inflammation, but a pseudo-acne situation can occur as a result of the primary irritant dermatitis seen with many of the more effective topical therapies such as vitamin A acid and benzoyl peroxide[10]. This is particularly so early in treatment, and this apparent flare in the acne must be discussed with the patients, otherwise they will stop the treatment prematurely.

Topical induction by hyperkeratinization

In this section the hyperkeratinization of acne vulgaris will be discussed, as will certain well-recognized clinical entities such as cosmetic acne, pomade acne, chloracne, steroid acne, tar acne and acne detergicans.

There is no doubt that subjects with acne do have ductal hyper-keratinization. This is obvious clinically as blackheads and white-heads, and the amount of hyperkeratinization can be quantified. In 1972 Holmes, Williams and Cunliffe[11], using the surface biopsy technique[12], sampled follicular casts from the backs of subjects with various degrees of acne. Table 1 shows that there is an increase in the number of hairs coated with keratin-like material and the degree of coating was significantly related to the severity of the acne. Electron microscopy of the samples revealed multiple interlacing lamellae filled with lipid droplets.

Table 1 Percentage of hairs 'coated' with keratin ($\pm$ SEM) and degree of keratin coating ($m \pm$ SEM) in subjects with different degrees of acne. Patients with a greater degree of acne have more keratin at this site

	Percentage of hairs coated with keratin	Degree of keratin coating
Controls	18.7 ± 1.3	1.5 ± 0.1
Mild acne	28.5 ± 0.2	2.1 ± 0.3
Moderate and severe acne	35.1 ± 4.3	2.9 ± 0.7

There are few models for hyperkeratinization but undoubtedly the best is the rabbit ear model as introduced by Kligman and Katz in 1968[13]. In this technique comedogenic substances are placed on one ear of the rabbit with the control on the other ear. This model has demonstrated that many substances induce comedones. In particular it has been demonstrated that free fatty acids, especially oleic acid and squalene, are comedogenic. It was therefore postulated that these substances irritate the pilosebaceous duct lining as they pass through, and induce hyperkeratosis. The same animal model has demonstrated that other substances such as lanolin, petrolatum, certain vegetable oils and certain pure chemical substances such as butyl stereate and lauryl alcohol could also induce ductal hyperkeratosis. More recently Mills and Kligman[14] have extended this type of assay to man. The agent under test is placed on the back under occlusion for several weeks. The results are similar to those in the rabbit ear model but the rabbit ear model tends to give a higher comedone score.

Fatty acids are produced in the pilosebaceous duct by the lipolysis of sebaceous triglycerides by bacteria. The presence of these fatty acids would therefore suggest that bacteria were important early on in the induction of hyperkeratinization. However, ultrastructural work by Lavker, Leyden and McGinley[15] demonstrated that in some of the early comedones of prepubertal subjects there were very few or no bacteria, indicating that the initiation of comedogenesis is possibly unrelated to bacteria. Quantification of bacteria in the pilosebaceous ducts (Leeming, Holland and Cunliffe[16]) also showed that early comedones contain no bacteria. These authors biopsied the skin and separated the pilosebaceous ducts using 'Kellum's' technique[17]. They then removed the pilosebaceous units from the epidermis, homogenized the sample and examined it for bacteria. They carefully checked that the technique did not kill the bacteria and their studies amply demonstrated that 80% of normal follicles and 20% of early whiteheads and blackheads are totally free of bacteria.

Thus the early hyperkeratinization of acne is not wholly produced by bacteria but later, microbial induction through the production of fatty acids, may be important.

What then are the reasons for the initial hyperkeratinization of acne? It may be due to an end organ response of the pilosebaceous duct to circulating androgens; there is indirect evidence that androgens have a direct effect on ductal keratinization (Shuster, personal communication, 1982). It is also possible that lipids other than fatty acids, such as squalene and wax ester, also play an important role. It would be of value to know the lipid composition of individual follicles at various stages of their development and such a study could throw light on the morphogenesis of acne lesions.

Topical induction of acne by hydration

Shakespeare described kitchen wenches with acne. In World War II some of the service men from the UK were returned to England because of a flare of their acne in humid environments. The precise reason for this so-called 'hydration acne' is uncertain. Physiological studies measuring the size of the pilosebaceous duct have demonstrated that hydration of the skin with polythene occlusion or after sweating induced by a hot bath reduces the size of the pore. It is conceivable that after such an event there would be some functional obstruction of the duct and this might precipitate acne lesions[18]. Indeed, measurement of sebum excretion following hydration of the skin does demonstrate that there is initially some blockage and that thereafter there is an overshoot of the sebum to a level significantly greater than on control sites, indicating that hydration will interfere with the flow dynamics of the sebum[18].

Topical induction – certain clinical entities

In 1972 Plewig, Fulton and Kligman[8] demonstrated in a study of 735 Negroes that 70% of them applied pomades which induced a non-inflammatory acne. This problem is also seen in the United Kingdom, particularly in West Indians who very often continue to apply pomades made locally by their West Indian shopkeepers.

Kligman and Mills[19] also demonstrated that 33% of mature American females had non-inflamed lesions, particularly in the perioral area. We do see cosmetic acne in the UK and certain make-ups will induce acne, the lesions being mainly non-inflamed. Nevertheless in the United Kingdom, at least for certain in Leeds, there is far less cosmetic acne than in Philadelphia. There are several possible reasons for this; cosmetics may be different; low quantities of cosmetics may be used – one's impression is that many American women wear heavy long-use cosmetics compared to Leeds women. In Leeds we have fewer Negroes, and the environment in Leeds is cooler and less humid than in Philadelphia. Nevertheless we thought it worthwhile checking whether cosmetics played a major role in the persistence of acne. We investigated 139 subjects; the details are shown in Table 2. The severity of the facial grade was related to the duration of acne and not the length of time for which they had used cosmetics. The ratio of the acne on the face and chest was also recorded. The table shows that those subjects who had used cosmetics for greater than 25 000 h had no increase in the severity of their acne. The ages of these patients were not significantly different. If cosmetics played a significant role in mature acne one would expect that the ratio of acne on the face to chest would be greater in those who had used the cosmetics for longer, but this was not so.

Table 2 Lack of relationship between acne severity, acne duration and hours use of cosmetics

	Less than 10 000 h	Around 12 500 h	More than 25 000 h
No. of patients	68	20	21
Duration of acne (years)	5.7 ± 3.2	7.6 ± 3.8	8.8 ± 4.1
Facial grade	2.6 ± 1.1	1.9 ± 1.1	2.1 ± 1.0
Ratio of acne face/chest	2.6	1.65	2.25

Chloracne

Chloracne is usually due to the effect of halogenated hydrocarbons on the skin following some industrial incident[20]. The hydrocarbon acts on the skin directly, or indirectly following ingestion. The result is a non-inflammatory acne which may spread to other members of a family because of the very marked comedogenic nature of the drug. Systemic features may also occur, but sometimes cutaneous features only are evident.

Steroid-induced acne

Topical corticosteroids, especially the fluorinated steroids, do induce acne[21]. Sometimes the eruption is predominantly that of comedonal acne, but occasionally the lesions are of a more inflammatory nature. The mechanism of steroid acne is in part due to ductal hyperkeratinization[22].

Miscellaneous conditions

There have been several reports of localized acne occurring as a result of friction to the skin, for example, fiddler's acne[23], hippie acne and friction from clothing such as the well-fitting bulky clothes of American footballers, and beneath riding hats[24].

There is no doubt that hyperkeratinization producing non-inflamed lesions is a clinical feature of acne. The precise morphogenesis of inflamed lesions is still open to question. The earlier work of Kligman and Strauss suggested that all inflamed lesions were preceded by non-inflamed lesions. Recent work by Blanc and Cunliffe (unpublished observations) suggested that perhaps a third of inflamed lesions were not preceded by non-inflamed lesions.

TOPICAL REDUCTION IN ACNE

Topical reduction in sebum excretion rate

There is no satisfactory topical treatment of acne which reduces sebum excretion rate. Two studies have shown that antiandrogens applied topically will reduce sebum excretion but this is only in females, the effect is limited, and furthermore the effects are not clinically significant[25,26]. There are several reasons why antiandrogens are as yet topically ineffective. In males there is so much endogenous androgen. In females a change in local biosynthetic androgen pathways may eventually overcome the topically applied antiandrogen.

Topical reduction in microflora

In the United Kingdom one of the most widely used topical therapies is benzoyl peroxide. This is available in several concentrations and formulations and many detailed studies would be needed to decide which is the best of the available preparations. Some of these preparations are available just as benzoyl peroxide; others are in combination with compounds such as hydroxyquinolone and sulphur.

There is no doubt that benzoyl peroxide works well in acne, producing, by the end of 3 months, a 50% reduction in the total number of lesions. Both non-inflamed and inflamed lesions are affected. The preparation produces a primary irritant dermatitis in many people and this settles with continued use; an allergic contact reaction is uncommon[27].

A newer approach to the topical treatment of acne with anti-microbial therapy is the use of pro-drugs in which a non-active drug such as ethyl lactate is applied to the skin[28]. This is acted upon by bacterial lipases which convert the ethyl lactate to lactic acid; this in turn affects the microenvironment of the organisms and so reduces the viable activity of these bacteria.

In the last 7 years there has been a tremendous interest in the use of topical antibiotics in the treatment of acne in the UK. In the USA there are now six preparations available for commercial use, whereas there is only one commercially available in the UK – in the form of chloramphenicol. There is no doubt that topical antibiotics do work and that clindamycin is probably the superior, with erythromycin number two and topical tetracycline the least effective[29-30]. These drugs act by reducing the number of bacteria. Tetracycline and erythromycin are only bacteriostatic but clindamycin is bactericidal.

There is also controversy as to the safety of topical antibiotics[31]. Clinically in the USA there have been no, or very few, untoward reactions but the pros and cons of using topical antibiotics in acne have been well reviewed by Eady and colleagues[31] and this was summarized in a leading article in *Lancet*, also in 1982. In brief Eady's thesis was that one should not use topically antibiotics which are used orally. It is well known that topical antibiotics will induce resistance in many of the *Staphylococcus epidermidis* when applied to the skin of acne patients. *S. epidermidis* will also code for genetic resistance[33]. Furthermore it is likely that the antibiotic will be transferred, because of the large amounts applied to the skin, onto inanimate objects, such as towels and directly onto other members of the family and friends. The result therefore could be that after 4–5 years of topical antibiotic use in acne a widespread increase of resistant *S. epidermidis* with a transfer of resistance to *S. aureus*, not just for the antibiotic used but also to other antibiotics. There is therefore a need for a large comprehensive study to determine whether or not there is a risk in the long-term use of topical antibiotics in acne.

There is also a need for adequate comparative studies of topical antibiotics with oral antibiotics and with non-antibiotic substances such as benzoyl peroxide. The limited data that are available suggest that topical antibiotics are less effective than oral antibiotics, with one, possibly two, exceptions[30]. There is also evidence that erythromycin topically is marginally less effective than benzoyl peroxide[32].

Topical reduction in acne by reduction in inflammation

Benzoyl peroxide will reduce the inflammation of acne within 5 days[34]. Whether this is a bacterial effect or some action on complement or other mediators of inflammation is uncertain.

Topical reduction in comedones

Certain topical therapies do reduce non-inflamed lesions. Vitamin A acid produces a greater reduction in non-inflamed lesions than any other topical therapy[35]. Benzoyl peroxide does reduce non-inflamed lesions[36] and the value of topical antibiotics in this context is controversial.

Using the follicular biopsy technique of Marks and Dawber[12] it can be shown that certain topical preparations are more effective than others in reducing the number of follicular casts[14]. Vitamin A is the most active; 5% salicylic acid in 85% ethanol and 15% propylene glycol will produce a 40% reduction; 10% resorcinol in the same base will produce a 13% reduction, which is of the same order as benzoyl peroxide. The role of sulphur in either producing or reducing comedones is still equivocal but a study by Strauss et al.[37] supported the view that sulphur is not comedogenic.

The human follicular cast model for testing the anticomedogenicity of drugs is valuable but does not necessarily relate to the clinical scene. Benzoyl peroxide does reduce the non-inflamed lesions by 50%[36] but in this latter model a 10% reduction only is obtained. It should also be remembered that in clinical terms whiteheads are far more frequently seen than blackheads, and the follicular biopsy technique is not so good at removing whiteheads.

Choice of therapy

There are many problems here. Which topical preparation should be used, when should they be used, with what should they be used and for how long?

The personal choice of the author in order of preference is benzoyl peroxide, vitamin A acid, and topical antibiotics. Benzoyl peroxide is probably better tolerated than vitamin A acid; in certain centres in the United States vitamin A acid is preferred. Perhaps English skins are less tolerant to the irritant effects seen with both preparations.

There are very few studies indicating whether topical therapy should be given with oral antibiotics but personal observations support the use of both treatment modalities.

Topical therapy is not needed with oral retinoids but it would not seem unreasonable to use a product such as benzoyl peroxide in conjunction with oral antiandrogens. Oral antiandrogens, although hitting the main target for acne, the sebaceous gland, needs a little extra help initially and a drug such as benzoyl peroxide could have an added advantage by directly killing the bacteria.

Topical therapy should be used in conjunction with oral antibiotics, in patients with mild acne, and in those subjects whose acne has come under good control with oral therapy and in whom oral therapy has been discontinued.

CONCLUSION

There is no doubt that acne can be caused by topical agents. There is considerable debate as to whether the induction of ductal hyper-keratinization in acne vulgaris is due to the irritant effect of sebum directly, or indirectly, influenced by bacteria. Many chemicals, topically applied, such as chlorinated hydrocarbons, steroids, certain cosmetics and pomades will induce an acne which is mainly non-inflamed in appearance.

Topical treatment is undoubtedly valuable in acne. There is no satisfactory topical treatment which reduces sebum excretion. Most successful topical treatments influence acne by either reducing keratinization or the number of bacteria, and therefore indirectly or directly affecting inflammation.

Topical therapy should be used by itself in mild and mild-to-moderate acne. It should also be used in conjunction with oral antibiotics in most acne patients and alone after stopping oral therapy. Although individual choices do differ the personal preference of the authors, in order, are benzoyl peroxide, vitamin A acid and topical antibiotics.

References

1. Cunliffe, W. J. and Shuster, J. (1969). Pathogenesis of acne. *Lancet,* 1, 685–687
2. Plewig, G., Fulton, J. E. and Kligman, A. (1971). Cellular dynamics of comedo formation in acne vulgaris. *Arch. Dermatol. Forsch.,* 242, 12–16
3. Cove, J. H., Holland, K. T. and Cunliffe, W. J. (1980). Acne vulgaris: is the bacterial population size significant? *Br. J. Dermatol.,* 102, 277
4. Kersey, P., Sussman, M. and Dahl, M. (1980). Delayed skin test reactivity to Propionibacterium acnes correlates with severity of inflammation in acne vulgaris. *Br. J. Dermatol.,* 103, 651–655
5. Strauss, J. S., Kligman, A. and Pochi, P. E. (1962). The effect of androgens on the human sebaceous gland. *J. Invest. Dermatol.,* 39, 139–155
6. Marples, R. R. (1969). The effect of hydration on bacterial flora of the skin. In Maibach, H. I. and Hidlick-Smith, G. (eds.) *Skin Bacteria and their Role in Infection,* p. 33. (New York: McGraw-Hill)
7. Holland, K. T., Cunliffe, W. J. and Roberts, C. D. (1978). The role of bacteria in acne: a new approach. *Clin. Exp. Dermatol.,* 3, 253
8. Plewig, G., Fulton, J. E. and Kligman, A. (1972). Pomade acne. *Arch. Dermatol.,* 101, 580–584
9. King, K., Jones, D. H., Daltrey, D. C. and Cunliffe, W. J. (1982). A double-blind study of the effects of 13-cis-retinoic acid on acne, sebum excretion rate and microbial population. *Br. J. Dermatol.,* 107, 583–590
10. Olsen, T. G. (1982). Therapy of acne. *Med. Clin. N. Am.,* 66, 851–871
11. Holmes, R. L., Williams, M. and Cunliffe, W. J. (1972). Pilosebaceous duct obstruction and acne. *Br. J. Dermatol.,* 87, 827
12. Marks, R. and Dawber, R. P. R. (1971). Skin surface biopsy: an improved technique for the examination of the living layer. *Br. J. Dermatol.,* 98, 53
13. Kligman, A. and Katz, A. M. (1968). Pathogenesis of acne vulgaris – comedogenic properties of human sebum in the external ear canal of the rabbit. *Arch. Dermatol.,* 98, 53
14. Mills, O. M. and Kligman, A. M. (1982). A human model for assaying comedolytic substances. *Br. J. Dermatol.,* 107, 543–548
15. Lavker, R. M., Leyden, J. L. and McGinley, K. J. (1981). The relationship between bacteria and the abnormal follicular keratinization in acne vulgaris. *J. Invest. Dermatol.,* 77, 325–330
16. Leeming, J. L., Holland, K. T. and Cunliffe, W. J. (1982). Is there a role for bacteria in the initiation of acne vulgaris. Data presented at E.S.D.R. meeting, Amsterdam
17. Kellum, R. E. (1966). Isolation of human sebaceous glands. *Arch. Dermatol.,* 93, 610–612
18. Williams, M., Cunliffe, W. J. and Gould, D. (1974). Pilosebaceous duct physiology. 1. Effect of hydration on pilosebaceous duct orifice. *Br. J. Dermatol.,* 90, 1
19. Kligman, A. and Mills, O. M. (1972). Acne cosmetica. *Arch. Dermatol.,* 106, 843–850
20. Taylor, J. S. (1974). Chloracne: a continuing problem. *Cutis,* 13, 585
21. Plewig, G. and Kligman, A. M. (1973). Induction of acne by topical steroids. *Arch. Dermatol. Forsch.,* 247, 29
22. Kaidbey, K. and Kligman, A. (1974). Pathogenesis of topical steroid acne. *J. Invest. Dermatol.,* 62, 31–36

23. Peachey, R.D.G. and Matthews, C.N.A. (1978). Fiddler's neck. *Br. J. Dermatol.*, **98**, 669

24. Frank, S. (1974). Uncommon aspects of common acne. *Cutis*, **13**, 817–822

25. Simpson, N.B., Bowden, P.E., Forster, R.A. and Cunliffe, W.J. (1979). The effect of topically applied progesterone on sebum excretion rate. *Br. J. Dermatol.*, **100**, 687

26. Lyons, F. and Shuster, S. (1982). Sex difference in response of the human sebaceous gland to topical flutamide. *Br. J. Dermatol.*, **107**, 697

27. Cunliffe, W.J. (1981). *Acne.* Update Postgraduate Centre Series. Update Publications Ltd

28. Swanbeck, G. (1972). A new principle for the treatment of acne. *Acta Dermatovenereol.*, **52**, 406

29. Jones, E.L. and Crumley, A.F. (1981). Topical erythromycin vs. blank vehicle in a multiclinic acne study. *Arch. Dermatol.*, **117**, 551

30. Gratton, D., Raymond, G.P., Guertin-Larochelle, S., Maddin, S.W., Leneck, C.M., Warner, J., Collins, J.P., Gaudreau, P. and Bendl, B.J. (1982). Topical clindamycin versus systemic tetracycline in the treatment of acne. *J. Am. Acad. Dermatol.*, **7**, 50–53

31. Eady, E.A., Holland, K.T. and Cunliffe, W.J. (1982). Should topical antibiotics be used for the treatment of acne vulgaris? *Br. J. Dermatol.*, **107**, 235–246

32. Burke, B., Eady, E.A. and Cunliffe, W.J. (1983). Benzoyl peroxide versus topical erythromycin in the treatment of acne vulgaris. *Br. J. Dermatol.*, **108**, 199–204

33. Naidoo, J. and Noble, W.C. (1981). Transfer of gentamicin resistance between coagulase-negative and coagulase-positive staphylococci on skin. *J. Hygiene* (Cambridge), **86**, 183–187

34. Schutte, H., Cunliffe, W.J. and Forster, R.A. (1982). The short term effects of benzoyl peroxide lotion on the resolution of inflamed acne lesions. *Br. J. Dermatol.*, **106**, 91

35. Plewig, G. and Braun-Falco, O. (1975). Kinetics of epidermis and adnexa following vitamin A acid in the human. *Acta Dermatovenereol.*, **55** (suppl.), 86

36. Cunliffe, W.J., Dodman, B. and Ead, R. (1978). Benzoyl peroxide in acne. *Practitioner*, **220**, 479–481

37. Strauss, J.S., Goldman, P.H., Nacht, S. and Gans, E.H. (1978). A re-examination of the potential comedogenicity of sulphur. *Arch. Dermatol.*, **114**, 1340–1342

2
Unwanted Side-Effects from Topical Agents and Tests for Them

R. MARKS

The skin is not a canvas on which cosmeticians can indiscriminately paint a delectable youthful scene; neither is it a sheet of denim from which grease and filth can be removed by scrubbing with alkaline solutions or strong detergents. It is an efficient but vulnerable membrane that grudgingly allows a controlled exchange of substances between the delicate tissues within and the threatening external environment. Its vulnerability is increased by persistent or repeated intimate contact with a foreign material, which is why any form of topical application can prove harmful.

Virtually everything put on the skin, including water, can cause damage if contact is sufficiently close and prolonged[1]. It follows that attention must be given to cosmetics and toilet applications as well as pharmaceutical products for topical use, as similar toxicity problems may arise with all of them. Allergic contact dermatitis to lanolin looks similar regardless of whether the causative agent was a foundation cream, a lanolin-containing soap or a corticosteroid ointment with the compound as part of its formulation. In fact almost the same problems may be evident in less obvious industrial settings. The clothing industry is one such example, as dyes, waterproofing agents and other additives may cause toxic hazards.

The potential toxic side-effects from a topical application are either to the skin or to the organism as a whole after percutaneous penetration. The possibility of a systemic effect from an agent absorbed through the skin cannot be ignored, and dictates that whenever a novel material is to be used its complete toxicity profile must be known. However, here only the side-effects on the skin itself will be considered, as these are much more common. The problems of percutaneous penetration and transdermal penetration are dealt with elsewhere.

The commonest cutaneous side-effect is what has come to be termed 'primary irritant dermatitis', although no-one seems too certain as to what the term 'irritant' actually means. To save needless debate it seems reasonable to regard 'irritant' as synonymous with 'toxic' – another term that defies precise meaning. Most space will be devoted to this problem.

Allergic contact hypersensitivity is also a quite important side-effect from the use of topical agents. However, this is much less common than primary irritant dermatitis. It is nonetheless potentially more damaging for reasons that will be discussed a little later. Other cutaneous side-effects that must be considered are contact urticaria, phototoxicity, acneigenicity, disorders of pigmentation and neoplasia.

PRIMARY IRRITANT CONTACT DERMATITIS

The clinical pattern of this common disorder depends on the site and frequency of application and can vary from the subjective sensation of 'stinging' with material containing lactic acid to the gross skin erosion seen after application of 7% sodium lauryl sulphate under occlusion (Figure 1). However, in the majority of instances the pattern evoked is 'eczematous', i.e. is characterized by erythema, swelling and exudation in the short term and by scaling and skin thickening after it has been present for some time.

Light-skinned Caucasian subjects are much more susceptible to this type of reaction than darker individuals. In fact the propensity to chemical irritation is closely related to the susceptibility to sun sensitivity[2,3], which is again dependent on skin colour in large part. The basis of this 'supersensitivity' in light-complexioned folk is not certain. The density of stratum corneum of black-skinned individuals is greater than that of Caucasians[4] but whether this can be extrapolated to differences between Caucasian subjects, or can account for all the differences in reactivity to irritants, is uncertain.

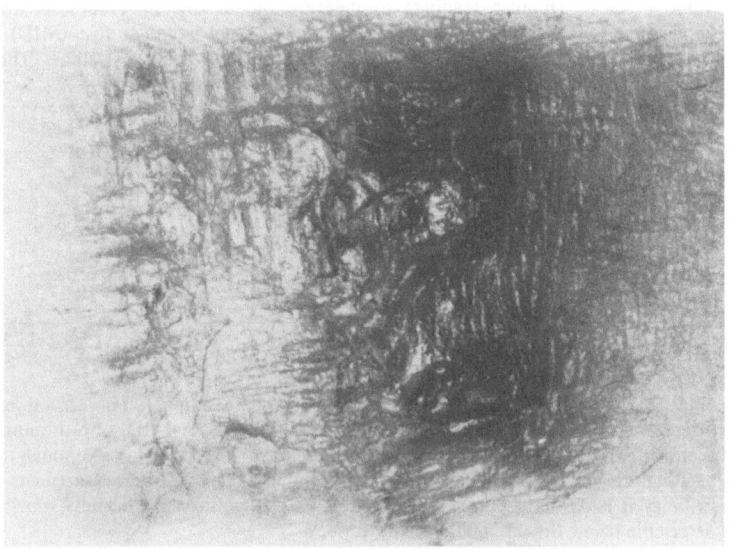

Figure 1 Crusted and eroded patch on upper arm after application of 7% sodium lauryl sulphate for 18 hours in volunteer subject

Curiously, older individuals are more resistant to chemical irritation than younger subjects[5,6]. Whether this is intrinsic to an ageing vasculature and reticuloendothelial system, or consequent on the increase in surface area of corneocytes in the elderly[7,8] and the changes in stratum corneum permeability which result, is unknown.

There is a pronounced regional hierarchy of sensitivity to irritants, with the face, neck and genitalia way out in front as the most easily irritated sites and the palms and soles the least. These differences may be in part due to differences in stratum corneum thickness.

An important practical issue is the additive effect of several mild irritants that are compounded together. Toxic effects do not obey an 'all-or-none' rule. Even when the dose of an irritant is below that needed to cause a clinical response, both structural and functional changes may be detected in the skin. We have recently demonstrated this using fractions of the minimal irritancy dose for anthralin and minimal erythema dose for ultraviolet light. The subclinical alterations in the skin were detected using laser Doppler measurements detecting changes in blood flow and ultrasound readings to measure

Table 1 Laser Doppler readings to measure blood flow in 4 subjects after application for 24 hours of increments of the minimal irritancy dose (MID) of dithranol in acetone to the skin of the back 24 hours after removal of patches. There is an increased blood flow detectable with even 0.1 of the irritancy dose

Doses	Mean ± SD
Control	0.17 ± 0.07
0.1 × MID	0.36 ± 0.30
0.5 × MID	0.81 ± 0.40
1.0 × MID	0.83 ± 0.40
2.0 × MID	1.06 ± 0.30
4.0 × MID	1.00 ± 0.30

Table 2 Ultrasound readings to measure skin thickness in 4 volunteer subjects after application for 24 hours of the minimal irritancy dose (MID) of dithranol in acetone to the skin of the back 24 hours after removal of the patches. Although this technique is not as sensitive as the laser Doppler method for measurement of irritancy it is clear that there is a dose-related change in skin thickness which is detectable below the minimal irritancy dose

Doses	Mean ± SD
Control	1.4 ± 0.1
0.1 × MID	1.4 ± 0.1
0.5 × MID	1.6 ± 0.4
1.0 × MID	1.7 ± 0.3
2.0 × MID	1.8 ± 0.2
4.0 × MID	2.1 ± 0.1

skin thickness (Tables 1 and 2). It is perhaps not surprising then that when two or more 'mild' irritants, which by themselves do not evoke a reaction, are formulated together, the mixture will cause an obvious irritant response.

The same consideration applies to repeated application of a mild irritant. A single application of a well-known therapeutically useful material – benzoyl peroxide, in the concentrations usually employed (3–10%) – rarely causes an irritant reaction. However, when the substance is used daily in the treatment of acne, redness and scaling develop in many patients after 3, 4 or 5 days.

If one concedes that this or that substance causes 'primary irritancy', have we described the reaction sufficiently or may each irritant reaction have particular characteristics of its own? There is some doubt whether all eczematous responses are essentially similar, or whether they only differ in severity and rate of development[9]. There can be little doubt that the overall reaction appears very similar, regardless as to whether alkali or dithranol irritancy or nickel allergy is to blame. Clearly the 'final pathway' is very similar with all toxic stimuli, but the mechanisms evoking it are probably not. There are clinical morphological differences between a positive patch test to nickel and an irritant patch test response to propylene glycol. These differences are not entirely dependent on whether allergic contact hypersensitivity or 'irritancy' are involved, as differences may be observed between reactions caused by different irritants – as, for example, between sodium lauryl sulphate and propylene glycol. Indeed I suspect that there are consistent clinical differences between reactions due to different contact allergens that are 'chemistry-dependent' rather than 'type of contact' dependent.

From the above it will be appreciated that many factors influence the development of irritant reactions. These factors include ethnic background, the degree of pigmentation, age, and body site in question. Obviously the concentration of the noxious substance, the frequency and intimacy of contact, the nature of the vehicle and the presence of other substances in the formulation will also profoundly influence the development of a primary irritant dermatitis. However, having set out these 'determinants', it should not be imagined that there are no others. The season of the year, previous exposure to irritants, and a history of an eczematous disorder may all influence the occurrence of irritant dermatitis as well.

ALLERGIC CONTACT DERMATITIS

This form of specific acquired hypersensitivity is now quite well characterized. It is mostly restricted to compounds of molecular weight greater than 500. However, there are few materials that have not sensitized someone at some time. For purposes of convenience it has become customary to talk of strong sensitizers, moderately strong, weak and non-sensitizers. On this basis one might classify the -caine group of local anaesthetics as strong sensitizers, neomycin as a moderately potent, and ethylene diamine as a weak sensitizer. Unfortunately there is no precision to these terms. A strong sensitizer may be expected to sensitize more than 3 or 4% of the population, a moderately strong sensitizer some 1 to 4%, and a weak sensitizer anything from 0.01 to 1%. Clearly when one is dealing with 'non-essential' topical agents, even a weak sensitizer is completely unacceptable.

Most industrial concerns have recognized this in recent years and now the number of cases of allergic contact dermatitis (ACD) due to cosmetics and toiletries is really very small – especially when one considers the volume sold of these articles. This (more or less) happy state of affairs is due to the selection of non-sensitizing substances for inclusion in products. Of course it does not prevent ACD from occurring in a few unfortunate subjects, and it is no comfort to these individuals to be told that their itchy, uncomfortable and unsightly rash is quite uncommon.

From the dermatologist's point of view the diagnosis of ACD to a cosmetic product can be quite a challenge. It may require an extremely painstaking history-taking session; something that is very difficult to do in a busy skin clinic. Identification of the allergen may also be difficult. More often than not the culprit allergen is not in the 'standard tray' of 20 allergens used by most dermatology departments in their screening battery. There are then several things that the dermatologist should do. The first is to ask the patient to bring all her (or his) cosmetics and toiletry products into the clinic so that they can be applied 'as is' in routine occlusive patch tests. Cleansing products and agents such as depilatories, perming materials and anything else that may be a strong primary irritant must be diluted before application (1 in 10 is usually adequate). If this procedure reveals a positive reaction, the clinician should then enquire from the company as to the composition of the offending material, so that the unfortunate individual can be advised not to use anything containing the chemical to which he or she is sensitive. If, as so frequently is the case, the application of the patient's cosmetics has drawn a blank, there are two other diagnostic manoeuvres that are worth pursuing. The first is to apply test patches of a battery of the more common sensitizers used in cosmetics[10]. These are 'pure' substances of the 'right' concentrations in the 'right' vehicle and are more likely to elicit a positive reaction. The second is to determine from the distribution of the rash which of the cosmetics is most likely to be involved and ask the patient to apply it (or them, if there is more than one) in the way that he or she normally does. This type of test in controlled circumstances may reveal sensitivities that are not evident from routine patch tests. It may be kinder to avoid this 'faithful' type of use test and apply the material to the forearm two or three times per day in an 'open patch test'. None of these tests should be contemplated while the original rash is still present or even in the period immediately after the rash has subsided. False-positive reactions are one consequence of not heeding this advice. Flare-up of the original rash if the responsible allergen is applied is the other possible result. Why the entire skin should be so 'irritable' and the affected site remain sensitive despite appearing normal is quite mysterious. The term used to describe this state of affairs is 'the angry back syndrome' and seems quite appropriate.

Before leaving allergic contact dermatitis and its diagnosis it has to be said that patch testing may seem a satisfying and simple procedure but if improperly performed can cause awful confusion. False-positives, false-negatives, sensitization to new agents and flare-ups of the eczema are some of the pitfalls that may be encountered. There is extensive information available on the pathogenetic mechanisms involved in allergic contact dermatitis as well as on its diagnosis, and for more detailed information the reader is referred to one of the monographs devoted to the topic[11,12].

OTHER TYPES OF REACTION FROM TOPICALLY APPLIED SUBSTANCES

The small amount of space to be devoted to these reactions is not a reflection on their interest or importance. It is merely a result of there being limited space and the need to concentrate on the most frequently encountered clinical problems.

ACNEIGENICITY

Many mineral oil containing preparations have the regrettable tendency to evoke an acneiform reaction. Such reactions are probably most likely in subjects who are anyway prone to acne, but it is by no means confined to them. The lesions produced are comedones and small papules or pustules, and larger, more inflamed lesions are

uncommon. This unfortunate side-effect of topical preparations has
been described as 'acne cosmetica'[13], 'pomade' acne[14], and 'fringe' or
'pop' acne[15]. The last describes the results of the use of oily hair preparations on the forehead skin. The acneiform reaction is probably
very much more common than believed, probably because it is usually
only a minor inconvenience rather than a dramatic and devastating
problem.

Contact urticaria

It is only in recent years that recognition has been given to this
unwanted side-effect of applications to the skin. Essentially the term
embraces weal and flare reactions developing within 1 hour of
contact. We are all aware of nettle plants causing an itchy, stinging
weal, but the reactions that occur in a substantial number of folk after
skin contact with common food additives such as benzoic acid,
cinnamic acid and cinnamic aldehyde are unrecognized. These reactions uncommonly spread outside the site of contact but certainly
can do so – and even produce unpleasant systemic reactions. Contact
reactions of the type referred to are not mediated by immunological
mechanisms. However, certain types of contact urticaria do appear to
have an immunological basis and these are not uncommon in atopic
subjects. Applications of egg, fruits or other foods elicit an urticarial
reaction in an appreciable number of such patients. The subject is well
reviewed by Cronin[16] and by Krogh and Maibach[17].

Light-induced dermatoses

Some materials when applied to the skin produce a dermatitis reaction
only after exposure to solar irradiation. Probably the most notorious
episode of phototoxicity due to topical applications concerns the
halogenated salicylanilides, used for their antimicrobial (and
deodorant) properties. Tetrachlorsalicylanilide (TCSA) (and similar
compounds) were used in soaps and produced unpleasant dermatitis
in the exposed areas. In some instances (as with TCSA) an immunological mechanism may be involved (photo-allergic) and in others the
reaction is more predictable and is termed phototoxic. The psoralens

are good examples of compounds that may cause phototoxic reactions. Although theoretically a reaction should develop in everyone exposed to the phototoxic substance after exposure to sunlight, this may not always be the case. Differences in percutaneous penetration and in the dose of UVR of the appropriate wavelength account for some of the variability. The chemical mechanisms of phototoxicity are complex[18].

Disturbances of pigmentation

Areas of hypopigmentation and/or hyperpigmentation may occur at sites of inflammation of the skin regardless of the cause, and minor degrees are quite common after eczema or psoriasis. This is due to damage to keratinocytes with liberation of the pigment into the dermis, or melanocyte dysfunction occurring in the course of the inflammatory reaction. Occasionally melanocyte hyperplasia occurs in the course of a hypertrophic eczematous process, resulting in hyperpigmentation.

Areas of pigmentation over the neck and sides of the face have been described due to photosensitization to Bergapten in oil of Bergamot. This 'Berloque dermatitis' occurs after an episode of dermatitis following application of eau de Cologne (containing oil of Bergamot).

More specific damage to the melanocyte cells occurs due to exposure to certain quinones, particularly monobenzyl ether of hydroquinone (MHQ) and paratertiary butyl phenol (PTBP). This has been a problem for workers in the rubber industry where outbreaks of a vitiligo-like disorder occurred. Interestingly the PTBP-induced depigmentation may have been caused by absorption of the compound by ingestion, inhalation or percutaneous penetration rather than by direct contact[19].

Neoplastic disease

As the development of neoplastic disease following topical application is considerably delayed compared to any other of the complications of topical preparations, this topic is intrinsically more difficult to describe and guard against. This is especially so as the process of carcinogenesis is multistage, and compounds may initiate the process, promote it or do both (complete carcinogens). Dimethylenbenz-anthracene, for example, is a 'complete carcinogen' and is used topically to induce papillomas and carcinomas on the skin of mice, whereas the phorbol esters (such as TPA) are tumour promoters.

Not unnaturally, there has been considerable concern over the possibility that products containing tars may be 'carcinogenic'. Tars result from the destructive distillation of coal and wood and contain literally thousands of phenolic, naphthalene- and anthracene-like compounds, some of which are potent carcinogens. The tars have been used for very many years for the treatment of a variety of skin disorders, notably psoriasis and eczema. There is no doubt that some tars can be shown to be carcinogenic in animal models and that human skin cancers can result from accidental contact over many years with soot or pitch, resulting in scrotal cancer in chimney sweeps and pitch warts in those working with this material. Nonetheless, the development of skin cancer from the use of tars used therapeutically is much less certain. Some studies appear to show that the risk of developing such neoplastic lesions in patients who have used these compounds over many years is extremely small – if present at all[20].

Dithranol used in the treatment of psoriasis can be shown to be mutagenic in the Ames test, and seems to be a tumour-promoter in some animal models. Once again, however, the risk of the development of skin cancer in treated patients seems to be negligible. Suspicion has even fallen on white soft paraffin, derived from distillation of oil. This product is also a complex mixture of organic compounds, some of which can be shown to be carcinogenic. Luckily there appears to be virtually no evidence that this has been responsible for any neoplastic lesions in man.

Another product that has caused concern is the dye, paraphenylene diamine, used to colour hair. However, as the major hazard appears to be due to percutaneous penetration and systemic absorption of the compound, this will not be considered further here.

Clearly the potential carcinogenicity of topically applied substances must always be carefully considered – especially with regard to new compounds. However, skin cancer as a result of application of currently used materials does not seem to constitute an appreciable hazard.

TESTING FOR TOXICITY OF TOPICALS

All products that come into contact with the skin should be free of toxicity. Whether the substance in question is a pharmaceutical agent designed for the treatment of skin disease, a cosmetic or an applicance of some sort, the same considerations apply. When the product is a powerful drug that can provide a striking benefit then a 'degree of toxicity' may be allowable. For example, the potential to cause some irritation of the skin may be permissible in a cream that helps clear psoriasis. It depends on that difficult-to-quantify parameter – the risk/benefit ratio. Regardless of this type of exception it behoves all manufacturers to take every possible measure to ensure that their products cause no harm. This involves monitoring for toxicity with reliably predictive tests. The same degree of care is required for products that contain well-characterized substances that are on various approved lists, although preliminary screening in animals or *in vitro* may not be required. It must be remembered that the rate and degree of skin penetration of a substance may well alter in a new formulation and that the minor toxicities of compounds can summate to produce a clinically apparent toxic reaction. Virtually all new topical agents should be assessed for irritancy, sensitization and phototoxicity. Cosmetics and toiletries may also need to be evaluated for acneigenicity, especially if they have a high oil content (particularly mineral oil).

TEST PROTOCOLS

Testing for irritancy

The traditional Draize tests on rabbit eyes[21] or shaved rabbit skin[22] are not sufficiently predictive for weak irritants[23]. Although animal testing performed in parallel with human tests gives broadly similar results the 'rank ordering' of irritants is not always the same. Because of this, and ethical, political and financial considerations, there can be little doubt that for 'finished products' human volunteer panel tests are more appropriate. The particular format of the test depends to some extent on the type of product to be tested. Most cosmetics and pharmaceutical preparations are best investigated in a repeat insult patch test, in which the material is placed in occlusive contact with the skin for 48 hour periods on several occasions at the same site. The test site is examined after each patch removal and scored on an arbitrary scale. Our own practice is to have panels of from 30 to 60 normal volunteer subjects of various skin types and to repeat the applications six times in 2 weeks. The various factors than can influence this type of study have been reviewed on several occasions recently[2,3,24].

Cleansing and detergent products cannot be tested in this straightforward way as they would be scored as moderately strong irritants. Two other tests have been proposed[25]: the antecubital fossa and face wash test and the soap chamber test. The latter has proved quite satisfactory in our hands and is the one that we routinely recommend. Depilatories and antiperspirants are also unsuitable for the routine repeat insult tests. Clearly the former would be strongly irritant and the only type of test would seem to be a use type test. A panel of volunteer subjects should use the material to depilate a small area of forearm skin first and then if this causes no problems, proceed to test small area of facial skin. Similar considerations apply to testing antiperspirants.

The testing of deeply coloured materials and stains presents a difficulty as reading and assessing erythema at the patch test sites becomes difficult. In these instances an instrumental technique can be used. We have employed simple thermometry to detect anthralin irritancy[26] and this seemed quite satisfactory. We have also used ultrasound and caliper measurement of skin thickness at the test sites[27] and others have employed the laser Doppler method for assessment of skin blood flow[28]. Thermographic methods have also been employed to detect positive responses to test materials[29]. However, the 'hardwear' required for this type of evaluation is complex and expensive, and it seems unlikely that this can be routinely used.

Instrumental techniques have much to commend them, even for assessment of non-staining substances, for two reasons. Firstly it removes the subjectivity in the detection of erythema. It may seem a simple business to detect when a patch is red and when it is not, but those who are involved in the reading of patch tests know that differences in lighting and the variegate nature of normal skin colour make it very difficult at times. Secondly there is value in the ability to measure the degree of response to a particular irritant. Certainly the 'all-or-none' detection of irritancy[30] will suffice in most instances but the determination of a particular dose–effect relationship may be important with some materials.

It has been suggested that 'compromising' the test site by 'adhesive tape stripping' or 'light scarification' makes the detection of irritancy a more sensitive process[31]. This may be so, but the removal of the normal horny layer barrier makes the tests too sensitive, in our estimation, and can give rise to false-positives.

Testing for sensitization

Detection of the capacity of a compound to cause allergic contact hypersensitivity is intrinsically more difficult than assessment of its potential for irritation. A major problem is the lack of criteria in defining what is acceptable and what is not. Obviously strong and moderately strong sensitizing agents must be avoided unless there is some very important 'benefit' to be obtained from the product that is not obtainable by other means. The difficulty arises in defining a weak sensitizer and knowing whether to use it in a topical formulation as so many substances can cause sensitization occasionally.

Although human volunteer tests are ideal for testing for irritancy they are less than perfect for detection of weak sensitizers. It has been suggested that there are ethical problems to such tests, as the testing itself can produce permanent sensitivities. The interpretation of such tests also requires caution. Negative results in a panel of 100 volunteers only means that under the conditions of the test the substance(s) under investigation have not sensitized 1% of the panel. But would the substance(s) sensitize 0.5, 0.25 or even 0.05% of the population to be exposed? Clearly there are major practical difficulties to testing larger groups of volunteers, yet larger numbers are needed to give the safety assurances necessary.

Animal tests have been devised that appear to be adequately predictive for strong and moderately strong sensitizers and helpful (but by no means perfect) for weak sensitizers. When new substances are included in formulations it would seem prudent to arrange for such a test as the first step. The most useful of these tests is the Magnusson–Kligman maximization test in guinea pigs[32]. This includes injections of Freund's adjuvant but topical application of the substances tested. The Buhler test[33] and the Klecek open epicutaneous test[34] both attempt to mimic the usual route of sensitization. The most sensitive of these animal tests reputedly is the Magnusson–Kligman protocol and positive results in this test have been categorized by Marzulli and Maibach[35] as 0–8% (weak), 9–28% (mild), 29–64% (moderate), 65% (strong) and 81–100% (extreme).

Formulations that contain well-known and much-used compounds, or newer compounds that are negative or very weakly sensitizing in the guinea pig maximization test, should be tested in a repeat insult in a panel of human volunteers for a final reassurance.

Phototoxicity and photosensitization

This is a complex topic, fraught with pitfalls for the unwary. Unlike irritancy and contact allergy, *in vitro* tests are available, although they do not succeed in identifying all known compounds that cause problems after light exposure. The candida killing test[36], the photo-haemolysis tests[37], and the histidine degradation test[38] are all useful for certain classes of compounds that exert their toxic action via different mechanisms. *In vitro* tests and their significance are reviewed by Addo *et al.*[39].

Tests in animals and man require xenon arc sources (solar simulator) for the best results although the action spectrum of the large majority of compounds that cause light-induced dermatoses is in the long (UVA) wavelength portion of the ultraviolet spectrum. Numerous tests have been described for both phototoxicity and photo contact allergy, and this is not the place for a detailed review of the advantages and disadvantages of each. Suffice to say that the modification of the human repeat insult test in which the test site is irradiated subsequent to each application, as described by Kaidby[40], and the newer guinea pig test described by Harber *et al.*[41] seem the best available.

Acneigenicity

Some workers distinguish between 'comedogenicity' and 'pustulo-genicity' as different mechanisms seem to be involved. The rabbit ear test for comedogenicity may be too sensitive, giving rise to false-positives, and Strauss[42] has proposed a similar test in man. An occlusive test in man for pustulogenicity has also been proposed.

CONCLUSION

None of the test systems presently available is ideal. They are beset by the problems of sensitivity and reproducibility as well as by ethical, political and financial dilemmas. Nonetheless, testing for topical toxicity is required for all substances that come into contact with the skin. Care must be taken to choose the most appropriate tests and to interpret the results that are generated with circumspection.

References

1. Kligman, A. M. (1982). Assessment of mild irritants. In Frost, P. and Horwitz, S. N. (eds.) *Principles of Cosmetics for the Dermatologist.* (St Louis: C. V. Mosby Co.), p. 265
2. Kligman, A. M. (1982). Assessment of mild irritants. In Frost, P. and Horwitz, S. N. (eds.) *Principles of Cosmetics for the Dermatologist.* (St Louis: C. V. Mosby Co.), pp. 265–273
3. Marks, R. and Kingston, T. (1984). Acute skin toxicity reactions in man: Tests and mechanisms. *Food Chem. Toxicol.* (In press)
4. Weigand, D. A., Haygood, C. and Gaylor, J. R. (1974). Cell layer and density of negro and caucasian stratum corneum. *J. Invest. Dermatol.,* **62,** 563–568
5. Grove, G. L., Duncan, S. and Kligman, A. M. (1982). Effect of ageing on the blistering of human skin with ammonium hydroxide. *Br. J. Dermatol.,* **107,** 393–400
6. Hamami, I., Black, D. and Marks, R. (1984). A comparison of skin response to mechanical and chemical trauma. Abstract of paper read at 14th Annual Meeting of European Society for Dermatological Research, Amsterdam, May
7. Grove, G., Lavker, R. M., Holzle, E. and Kligman, A. M. (1981). Use of non-intrusive tests to monitor age associated changes in human skin. *J. Soc. Cosmet. Chem.,* **32,** 15–18
8. Plewig, G. and Marples, R. R. (1970). Regional differences of cell sizes in human stratum corneum, Part II. Effects of age and sex. *J. Invest. Dermatol.,* **54,** 19–23
9. Cronin, E. (1980). *Contact Dermatitis.* (Edinburgh: Churchill Livingstone), pp. 29–31
10. Cronin, E. (1980). *Contact Dermatitis.* (Edinburgh: Churchill Livingstone), ch. 4, pp. 93–170
11. Fisher, A. A. (1973). *Contact Dermatitis.* (Philadelphia: Lea & Febiger)
12. Cronin, E. (1980). *Contact Dermatitis.* (Edinburgh: Churchill Livingstone)
13. Plewig, G., Fulton, J. E. and Kligman, A. M. (1970). Pomade acne. *Arch. Dermatol.,* **101,** 580

14. Kligman, A.M. and Mills, O.H. (Jnr) (1972). Acne cosmetica. *Arch. Dermatol.*, **106**, 843
15. Bowyer, A. (1965). Fringe or 'pop' acne. *Br. Med. J.*, **2**, 1548
16. Cronin, E. (1980). *Contact Dermatitis*. (Edinburgh: Churchill Livingstone), pp. 24–29
17. Krogh, G. von and Maibach, H. (1982). The contact urticaria syndrome 1982. In Kligman, A.M. and Leyden, J.J. (eds.) *Safety and Efficacy of Topical Drugs and Cosmetics*. (New York: Grune & Stratton), ch. 16, pp. 249–267
18. Kornhauser, A., Wamer, W., Giles, A. and Szabo, G. (1982). Mechanisms of light induced dermal toxicity. In Frost, P. and Horwitz, S.N. (eds.) *Principles of Cosmetics for the Dermatologist*. (St Louis: C.V. Mosby Co.), ch. 30, pp. 244–258
19. Cronin, E. (1980) *Contact Dermatitis*. (Edinburgh: Churchill Livingstone), p. 870
20. Maughan, W., Muller, S., Perry, H. *et al.* (1980). *J. Am. Acad. Dermatol.*, **3**, 612–615
21. Draize, J.H. (1959). Appraisal of the safety of chemicals in foods, drugs and cosmetics. In *Dermal Toxicity*, Austin, 1959, Association of Food and Drug Officials of the United States, Texas State Department of Health
22. Draize, J.H., Woodard, G. and Calvary, H.O. (1944). Methods for the study of irritation and toxicity of substances applied topically to the skin and mucous membranes. *J. Pharmacol. Exp. Ther.*, **82**, 377–389
23. Kligman, A.M. (1982). Assessment of mild irritants. In Frost, P. and Horowitz, S.N. (eds.) *Principles of Cosmetics for the Dermatologist*. (St Louis: C.V. Mosby Co.), ch. 33, pp. 265–273
24. Marks, R. (1983). Testing for cutaneous toxicity. In Balls, M., Riddell, R. and Worden, A. (eds.) *Animals and Alternatives in Toxicity Testing*. (New York: Academic Press)
25. Frosch, P.J. (1982). Irritancy of soaps and detergent bars. In Frost, P. and Horowitz, S.N. (eds.) *Principles of Cosmetics for the Dermatologist*. (St Louis: C.V. Mosby Co.), ch. 1, pp. 5–12
26. Kingston, T. and Marks, R. (1983). Irritant reactions to dithranol (anthralin) in normal subjects and psoriatic patients. *Br. J. Dermatol.*, **108**, 307–313
27. Kingston, T., Hamami, I. and Marks, R. (1984). A quantitative comparison of the irritancy of pure anthralin and Dithranol BP. *Arch. Dermatol. Res.* (In press)
28. Nilsson, G.E., Otto, U. and Wahlberg, J.E. (1982). Assessment of skin irritancy in man by Laser Doppler flowmetry. *Contact Dermatitis*, **8**, 401–406
29. Mustakallio, K.K. (1979). Irritation and staining by dithranol (anthralin) and related compounds. 1. Estimation with chamber testing and contact thermography. *Acta Dermato-Venerol.* (Suppl. 20), **105**, 64–67
30. Kligman, A.M. and Wooding, W.M. (1967). A method for the measurement and evaluation of irritants on human skin. *J. Invest. Dermatol.*, **49**, 78–94
31. Frosch, P.J. and Kligman, A.M. (1977). The chamber scarification test for assaying irritancy of topically applied substance. In Drill, V.A. and Lazar, P. (eds.) *Cutaneous Toxicity*. (New York: Academic Press)
32. Magnusson, B. and Kligman, A.M. (1970). *Allergic Contact Dermatitis in the Guinea Pig: Identification of Contact Allergens*. (Springfield, III: Charles C. Thomas)
33. Buhler, E.V. and Griffith, F. (1975). Experimental skin sensitization in the guinea pig and man. In Maibach, H. (ed.) *Animal Models in Dermatology*. (Edinburgh: Churchill Livingstone)

34. Klecak, G., Geleick, H. and Frey, J. R. (1977). Screening of fragrance materials for allergenicity in the guinea pig. I. Comparison of four testing methods. *J. Soc. Cosmetic Chem.,* **28**, 53–59

35. Marzulli, R. N. and Maibach, H. I. (1977). Allergenicity rating. In Marzulli, R. N. and Maibach, H. I. (eds.) *Advances in Modern Toxicology,* Vol. 4: *Dermatotoxicology and Pharmacology.* (Washington, DC: Hemisphere)

36. Kagan, J., Gabriel, R. and Reed, S. A. (1980). Alpha-terthienyl, a non-photo-dynamic phototoxic compound. *Photochem. Photobiol.,* **31**, 465

37. Frain-Bell, W., Hetherington, A. and Johnson, B. E. (1979). Contact allergic sensitivity to chrysanthemum and the photosensitivity dermatitis and actinic reticuloid. *Br. J. Dermatol.,* **101**, 491–501

38. Weil, L. (1965). On the mechanism of the photo-oxidation of amino acids sensitized by methylene blue. *Arch. Biochem. Biophys.,* **110**, 57–68

39. Addo, H. A., Ferguson, J., Johnson, B. E. and Frain-Bell, W. (1982). The relationship between exposure to fragrance materials and persistent light reaction in the photosensitivity dermatitis with actinic reticuloid syndrome. *Br. J. Dermatol.,* **107**, 261–274

40. Kaidby, K. (1982). Assessment of topical photosensitizers in humans. In Kligman, A. M. and Leyden, J. J. (eds.) *Safety and Efficacy of Topical Drugs and Cosmetics.* (New York: Grune & Stratton), ch. 13, pp. 213–220

41. Harber, L. C., Armstrong, R. B., Walther, R. R. and Ichikawa, H. (1982). Current status of predictive animal models for drug photoallergy and their correlation with humans. In Kligman, A. M. and Leyden, J. J. (eds.) *Safety and Efficacy of Topical Drugs and Cosmetics.* (New York: Grune & Stratton), ch. 10, pp. 177–191

42. Strauss, J. S., Goldman, P. H., Nacht, S. and Gars, E. H. (1978). Re-examination of potential comedogenicity of sulfur. *Arch. Dermatol.,* **114**, 1340

3
Psychorheology of Topical Applications

M. I. BARNETT

In the preparation of semi-solid products for application to the skin it is not too difficult to arrange the formulation to give particular types of rheological behaviour. This is achieved by variation of the components so that plasticity, pseudoplasticity and thixotropy may be obtained in varying degrees. It is also relatively easy to reproduce the rheological characteristics of a successful product firstly by interpreting and then by producing a facsimile of the formulation. The real problem to the formulator is to achieve a product that has the same 'skin feel', and hence the same acceptability, to the user.

Acceptability is not a definable term because of subjective variations in interpretation; a property that is acceptable to one person may not be acceptable to another. The acceptance or rejection of a topical application by a user is influenced by various properties of the product referred to by Barry and Grace[1] as the textural profile. This profile includes such parameters as appearance, odour, extrudability where applicable, initial sensations on contact with the skin, spreading properties, tackiness or stickiness, and the residual feel of the skin after the application of the product, e.g. smoothness or greasiness. If the initial organoleptic properties are acceptable, then the topical application procedure was described by Barry and Grace as being in four parts: (1) removal of the preparation from its container, (2) the initial sensation on the skin, (3) the sensations during spreading and (4) the final impressions due to the residue of the application on the skin. Ultimately the acceptance or rejection of a skin product by a user is influenced almost entirely by the feel of the product on the skin, so that whatever rheological parameters have been measured in the development and stability testing of the product, only those that relate to, or could be related to 'skin feel' will be important to the user.

ASSESSMENT OF SKIN FEEL IN RELATION TO THE APPLICATION OF SEMI-SOLIDS

Physical methods

The most common assessment is carried out by rubbing a product onto the skin; this is a dynamic assessment not only of the product but of the properties of the skin itself. Spreading of the product gives a wide range of stresses, and hence the fingers can perform a complete assessment for the individual. Examples of the applied shear rates can be found in the literature but their scientific basis is sometimes questionable. For instance, Henderson *et al.*[2] calculated the shear rates in the following way: an ointment was applied at four strokes/second, each stroke being 6 cm long and the average layer of ointment on the skin was given a thickness of 0.2 cm. The assumption was made that the layer of material in contact with the skin was stationary and the role of shear was calculated as $120 s^{-1}$. Barry and Meyer[3] obtained shear rates between $350 s^{-1}$ and $10^4 s^{-1}$ for the spreading of a variety of topical products whilst one of the more accurate assessments comes from a high-speed camera technique used by Mitsui *et al.*[4] who found maximum shear rates for the application of o/w cosmetic creams to be between 10^4 and $10^5 s^{-1}$. The prediction of the performance of a product from instrumental rheological characterization over a wide range of shear rates is therefore limited by interpretation of the actual shear rates involved during application to the skin.

The skin itself is rheologically complex; it demonstrates viscoelastic properties, which means that it will be elastic when quickly stretched by a small amount, but may flow slightly when deformed by greater forces for longer time periods. This means that any assessment of an application to the skin is also an assessment of the properties of skin itself. The viscoelastic behaviour of skin is shown diagrammatically in Figure 1; the 'springs' represent the elastic response of skin and the 'dashpots' represent the viscous response. The physical properties and measured values of these 'springs' and 'dashpots' have been estimated by Tregear[5].

Psychophysical methods

These are achieved by using test panels usually trained to define precise conditions such as smoothness, dryness, etc. These panels can

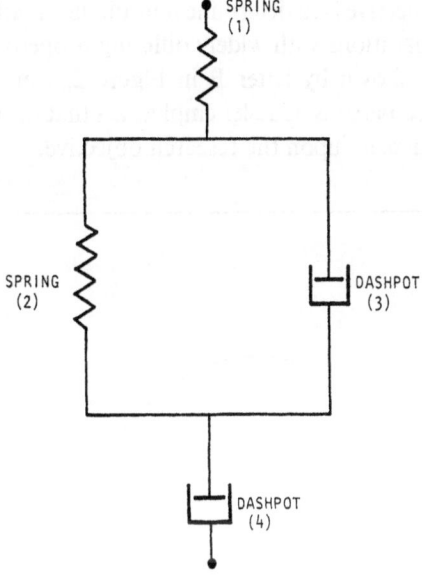

```
IMPOSED SHEAR STRESS:
                    SPRING (1) STRETCHES INSTANTLY
                          (2) STRETCHES MORE SLOWLY
                    WITH EXTENSION OF DASHPOT (4).

REMOVE STRESS:
                    SPRING (1) CONTRACTS TO ORIGINAL LENGTH.
                          (2) CONTRACTS SLOWLY - RETARDED
                              BY DASHPOT(3).

                    DASHPOT (4) UNAFFECTED BY REMOVAL OF
                                STRESS - RETURNS SLOWLY TO
                                ORGINAL POSITION.
```

Figure 1 Spring + dashpot model of creep behaviour of skin

often detect minor changes in a formulation and can actually be used in assessing a competitive product with a view to duplicating its skin feel. Cussler[6] provides a good example of this by using a hypothetical experiment for the evaluation of oiliness and in so doing gives an insight into the importance of trained panels. Cussler states that if the aim is to duplicate the oiliness of a preparation then a number of preparations of similar viscosity and apparently similar characteristics can best be evaluated by a trained test panel capable of precise distinctions. These points are shown by letter A on the curve in Figure 2. If, however, the objective is to determine how oiliness is affected by cream viscosity, preparations with widely differing properties would be tested and these, shown by letter B in Figure 2, can easily be perceived by untrained persons. Cussler emphasizes that the necessity for a test panel will depend upon the research objective.

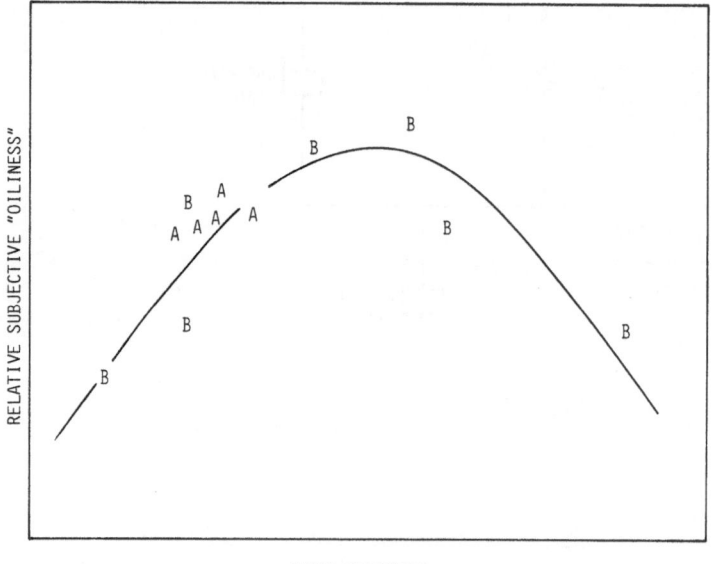

CREAM VISCOSITY

Figure 2   A hypothetical experiment for evaluating oiliness[6]

THE USE OF SCALES

The most common method of measuring subjective response is to give subjects a number of samples and invite them to grade them in a specific way. Some scaling systems can be biased by using inappropriate adjectives or limited descriptions assigned to letters or numbers. Some typical examples of scaling systems are:

Nominal Used to identify samples of equal texture.

Ordinal Presents samples to the user who is asked to express, for instance, which sample is the smoothest, next smoothest and so on.

Interval Assigning numbers to characterize a quality, e.g. 1 is poor, 2 is fair, 3 is good, etc.

Ratio One sample is chosen as a standard and others evaluated relative to it.

These scaling systems may then be interacted with rheological measurements to assess properties like 'spreadability' of a product[3].

DUPLICATING SKIN FEEL USING UNIVERSAL CURVES

Details of the construction, interpretation and use of universal curves are given by Cussler[6]. These curves are constructed by combining observations of subjective consistency with rheological measurements on a particular class of materials, e.g. o/w creams, w/o creams, or gels. Figure 3 shows the construction of a typical curve. Samples of a class of product are identified as having the same 'feel' and their complete rheological profiles are then drawn on a shear rate–shear stress diagram, the point of intersection of the two curves becoming the locus of the universal curve as for curves A and A'. Likewise B and B' have a similar feel and point of intersection and also form part of the universal curve. This process is repeated a number of times to produce the loci of the curve. Blocks representing the limits of experimental error are drawn around the intersections and the edges of the blocks are joined to give the area of the universal curve. Any two products whose rheological curves intersect within the confines of the universal curve area will have the same 'feel'. This concept could be an important way forward in the duplication of the skin feel of products.

This area of psychorheology or texture studies has been ignored, with one or two notable exceptions, for the last decade. The food industries are considerably more advanced than either the cosmetic or pharmaceutical industries, so perhaps it is time to re-address ourselves

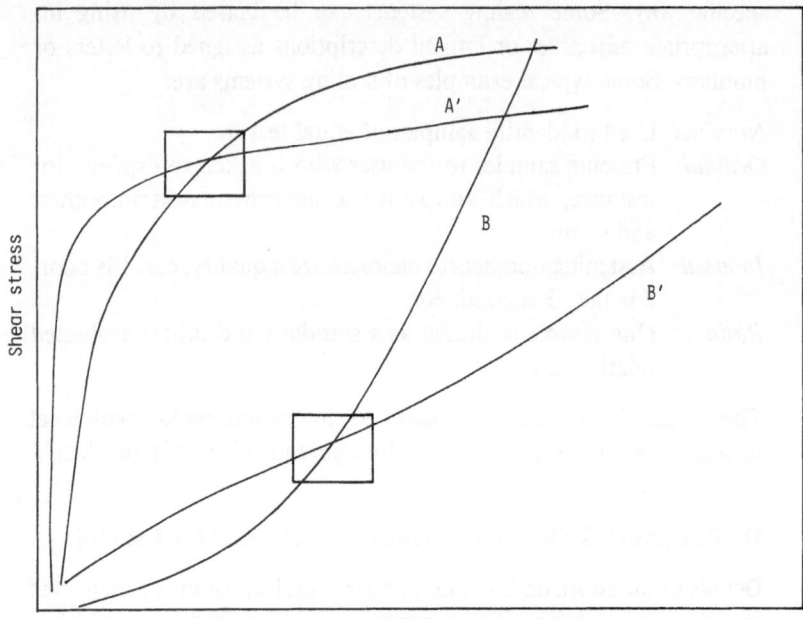

Figure 3 Construction of a universal curve

to the important question of what is acceptable to the patient/ consumer. A skin preparation with ideal drug release properties will not promote adherence to a treatment regimen without patient acceptability of the textural properties of that product.

References

1. Barry, B.W. and Grace, A.J. (1972). Sensory testing of spreadability: investigations of rheological conditions operative during application of topical preparations. *J. Pharm. Sci.*, **61**, 335-341
2. Henderson, N.L., Meer, P.M. and Kostenbauder, H.B. (1961). Approximate rates of shear encountered in some pharmaceutical processes. *J. Pharm. Sci.*, **50**, 788
3. Barry, B.W. and Meyer, M.C. (1973). Sensory assessment of spreadability of hydrophilic topical preparations. *J. Pharm. Sci.*, **62**, 1349-1354
4. Mitsui, T., Morosawa, K. and Otake, C. (1971). Estimation of the rate of shear encountered in topical applications of cosmetics. *J. Texture Stud.*, **2**, 339-347
5. Tregear, R.T. (1969). *J. Soc. Cosmet. Chem.*, **20**, 467
6. Cussler, E.L. (1978). *Cosmetic Science*, Vol. 1, pp. 117-152. (New York: Academic Press)

4
What do you do with a Topical Corticosteroid?

R. MARKS

The corticosteroids revolutionized treatment of chronic inflammatory disease in the 1950s and 1960s and since then topical preparations containing these agents have provided symptomatic relief for a vast number of patients. Although they have side-effects and theoretical disadvantages they are still immensely important as dermatological treatments.

Despite hydrocortisone being introduced in the early 1950s and potent topical agents such as betamethasone-17-valerate and fluocinolone acetonide being available some 10 years later, new topical corticosteroids are still being introduced to the market. The reasons for the continuing development of these compounds are complex. Part of the explanation may rest on the search for that elusive creature, the 'corticosteroid without side-effects', and part in what is euphemistically termed 'market pressure'. Regardless of the reasons, I have no doubt that more corticosteroids will be developed for topical use and this contribution concerns the means available for evaluation of the efficacy, potency and toxicity of these agents. A vast literature has accumulated on this topic and it is not my purpose to review it in detail, but more to select certain aspects for comment and hopefully to stimulate discussion.

EFFICACY AND POTENCY

There are considerable confusions concerning the use of these terms with regard to topical corticosteroids. 'Efficacy' is not the same as 'potency', although the two terms have close interrelationships. The term efficacy implies 'clinical efficacy' and may have very little to do with a drug's performance in human vasoconstrictor (VC) studies or its performance in animal models. To be 'clinically effective' an agent should act within an appropriately short time and continue acting for a sufficiently long period. Furthermore, it should suppress or eliminate the disease for which it is prescribed and should do so without producing unacceptable, unwanted side-effects.

The distinction between 'potency' and 'efficacy' may appear pedantic but may be important in deciding whether particular candidate compounds are developed or not. The McKenzie-Stoughton test[1] provides excellent data concerning potency but very little about clinical efficacy. Even with the modifications suggested by Barry and Woodford[2] in which the area under the curve of activity versus time supplies some information on the speed of VC effect (and the persistence of its action) or those of Clanachan et al.[3] who strongly supported standardized techniques, there is no certainty that a compound selected as the most potent will be effective and useful in the clinic. There are examples of corticosteroids that 'perform' well in human VC tests but have not been particularly useful in clinical tests. Whether this disparity can be explained on the basis of bioavailability of the compound from the finished formulations or on differences in the tissue distribution of the candidate substances because of particular partition coefficients, diffusional problems or special tissue affinities, remains to be seen.

It must also be remembered that human VC tests are performed on intact skin as opposed to clinical use in which the compounds are used on skin with a variably severe defect in the barrier function of the stratum corneum. Also, as the inflammatory change is suppressed, epidermal differentiation reverts to normal and the barrier is restored at a variable rate.

Because of the 'urge to economize' in British medicine and the laudable tendency to treat disease cautiously (if not conservatively), dermatologists (including the writer) have often diluted the more potent preparations when it was felt that the full potency was not required or that the risk of side-effects might be diminished. Whilst one can applaud the intention, it is by no means certain that the desired pharmacological end was being achieved by the simple act of dilution. In the first place dilution with anything other than the correct vehicle could well disrupt the release characteristics of the compound from the vehicle and make it less 'bioavailable'. Even worse, the act of dilution could dilute other essential components of the formulation, such as antimicrobial agents – making the preparation bacteriologically unsafe. But apart from these considerations it should be remembered that the action of a corticosteroid will depend on the degree of saturation of the receptor sites and the particular binding affinity of the corticosteroid in question[4,5]. It seems intrinsically unlikely that dilution of the corticosteroid preparation in the way practised will alter either of these, and hence is unlikely to alter the clinical efficacy to any great degree.

There is yet another 'pharmacophilosophical' issue as far as efficacy/potency is concerned. None of the common skin disorders that dermatologists are required to treat are the result of 'corticosteroid deficiency'. They are all the result of tissue injury triggering off complex cascades and ultimately producing a variable mix of mediators in the damaged tissue and the signs of inflammation. Clearly, all that any anti-inflammatory agent can do is to suppress the expression of the disease. This may give worthwhile symptomatic relief but is unlikely to alter the natural history of the disorder. Indeed there is some slight evidence that the signs of the disease return with increased vigour after the anti-inflammatory drug has been withdrawn. Certainly it has been suggested that pustular psoriasis is more likely after the treatment of ordinary plaque type psoriasis with corticosteroids[6].

Granted that the corticosteroids applied topically are 'potent' in suppressing inflammation in models, just how effective are they at altering the clinical expression of skin disease in practice? It may be thought a little 'late in the day', some 30 years after their inception, to ask such a fundamental question. However, I would remind readers that dilute hydrochloric acid was prescribed for many decades by dermatologists in the treatment of rosacea and was said to be 'effective', and there are other examples of even more outlandish treatments said during their fashion to be 'effective' but later discarded as useless. Topical corticosteroids were virtually the first dermatological agents to be introduced in elegant base vehicles and the first to be prettily presented and promoted. Could these factors have anything to do with their immediate acceptance and enormous commercial success? I believe that they could, and furthermore that these facts may have something to do with the continuing acclaim that the topical corticosteroids receive.

We have compared the action of corticosteroid preparations with those of bland agents on two occasions in patients with chronic hand eczema and found that there was no therapeutic benefit to be gained from the use of the 'active' preparation[7] (see Table 1). What can one learn from this sort of exercise? Firstly, that chronically inflamed skin may not respond as well as the various models tested suggest. Secondly, that bland emollient preparations are themselves useful agents, and finally, that a critical attitude to 'established therapies' may yield surprising information.

Many of the difficulties rest with the inadequacy of the models used and with the design of clinical trials for the evaluation of the topical corticosteroids. In general the models used are much more predictive for acute and self-limiting dermatoses than for persistent skin disorders. A variety of insults to human volunteer skin have been used over the years to evaluate the potential therapeutic effects of corticosteroids including the pyrexal test[8], the croton oil kerosene test[9], the poison ivy test[10], and an adhesive tape stripping test based on Pongsehirun et al.[11]. Although in broad general terms these tests produce a type of 'dermatitis' the reactions are all self-limiting. They do not really simulate spontaneous persistent skin diseases such as atopic dermatitis. The so-called 'psoriasis plaque test' of Dumas and Scholz[12] is an attempt to surmount this problem but in my view psoriasis should not be considered a target disease for the topical corticosteroids. Furthermore, the test evaluates the suppressive action of the compounds on a small area under rather artificial test conditions and not how the disease responds as a whole or how long it takes for the patch to recur.

This is not the place to bemoan the general standard of dermatological clinical trials. Nonetheless it is perhaps appropriate to suggest that when there are no criteria for the disease under investigation, no objective techniques for the assessment of any clinical response, and inadequate periods of evaluation, it is unlikely that even the most sophisticated statistics will produce anything other than confusion. Trials comparing the clinical efficacy of topical corticosteroids are very difficult to do and should not be undertaken lightly.

Table 1 Therapeutic effects of a bland emollient preparation and a corticosteroid preparation in patients with bilateral chronic hand eczema

| Clinical feature | Means and standard deviations for clinical scores (0 to 3 scale) at the start of the study and after 2 and 4 weeks | | | | | |
| | Initial evaluation | | Evaluation at week 2 | | Evaluation at week 4 | |
	UM*	BN 17-val† (0.025%)	UM*	BN 17-val† (0.025%)	UM*	BN 17-val† (0.025%)
Erythema	1.00 ± 0.50	1.05 ± 0.54	0.74 ± 0.77	0.80 ± 0.63	0.69 ± 0.74	0.79 ± 0.85
Scaling	1.30 ± 0.69	1.27 ± 0.65	0.98 ± 0.75	0.93 ± 0.66	0.76 ± 0.73	0.67 ± 0.75
Itching	1.50 ± 0.81	1.55 ± 0.94	0.69 ± 0.67	0.91 ± 1.04	0.54 ± 0.74	0.48 ± 0.73
Total	5.75 ± 2.43	6.10 ± 3.00	3.37 ± 3.69	3.69 ± 3.24	2.62 ± 2.67	3.09 ± 3.62

Hands were allocated at random to the treatments, and the study was conducted in double-blind fashion
* Unguentum Merck
† Betamethasone 17-valerate 0.025% ointment

UNWANTED SIDE-EFFECTS AND TOXICITY

Obviously there is the usual need to characterize the systemic (and local) toxicity of all new corticosteroids in the standard manner as for all new drugs. With corticosteroids, however, there are also some unwanted side-effects that need to be specially investigated. These are: (1) potential for suppression of the pituitary adrenal (PA) axis, and (2) ability to cause skin atrophy.

Pituitary–adrenal axis suppression

It is generally recognized that application of topical corticosteroids results in systemic absorption of the corticosteroid molecule and if sufficient of the compound is absorbed, suppression of the PA axis via the negative feedback mechanism occurs. Because of the dire clinical results that have been recorded (albeit rarely) from the use of potent and very potent corticosteroid preparations to large body areas for periods of more than a few days[13], registration bodies require information as to the degree of suppression caused by new preparations.

It must be realized that the tests employed to investigate the degree of PA axis suppression bear little relationship to the actual clinical use of the compound, and whether they are good predictors of potential hazard from PA axis suppression or not must be considered speculative. As has been pointed out elsewhere in this Symposium (see Ch. 9), percutaneous penetration through abnormal stratum corneum is much enhanced compared to normal skin. Thus when patients with inflammatory dermatoses are treated the flux of corticosteroid through the skin is initially greater, though as the condition improves the rate of penetration will decrease towards normal. In addition, in the chronic dermatoses patients use topical corticosteroids for long periods, but sometimes do so intermittently. It is just not possible to devise a protocol that adequately simulates the clinical usage under all conditions. However, manufacturers of corticosteroids and registration authorities require some information on the potential of a compound to produce PA axis suppression and are guided by data obtained from short-term challenge tests in normal volunteer subjects with healthy intact skin.

In a regimen that is often employed, 50 g of the corticosteroid preparation is applied daily to approximately 30% of the body area (25 g for 12 h under occlusion and 25 g after the occlusive dressing has been removed). The degree of suppression is assessed from the plasma cortisol levels. This value is assessed in early-morning 'fasting' samples taken for 5 days before the periods of application, during 5 days of application of the materials and for some days subsequent to the application (Figure 1). In this type of test the potent and moderately potent topical corticosteroids will induce some depression in the plasma cortisol level from the second day of application. This rapidly returns to pretreatment levels after the application stops. The

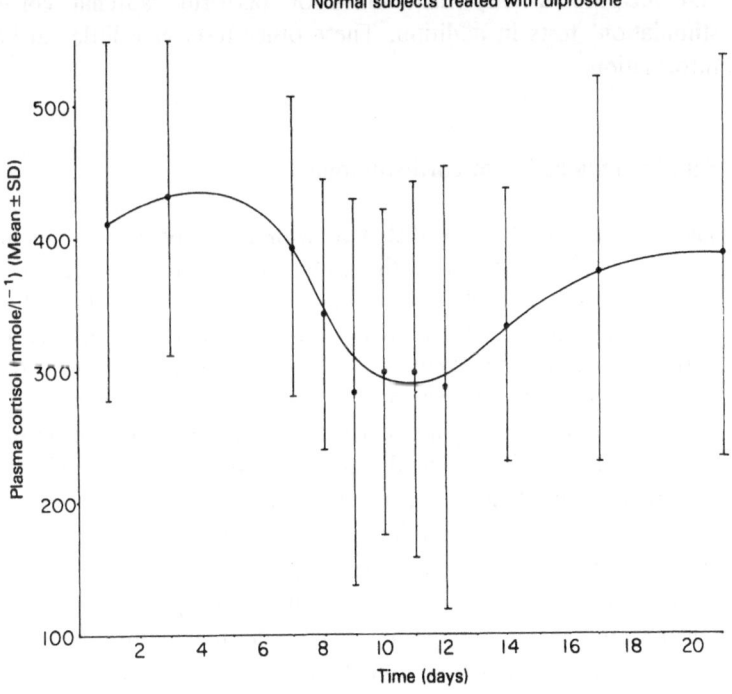

Figure 1 Eight normal volunteer subjects had Diprosone (betamethasone dipropionate 0.05%) applied daily – 30 g occlusively for 12 h and 30 g non-occlusively for 12 h – for a 5-day period from day 5. The plasma cortisol was estimated daily in early morning blood samples using a radioimmune assay technique

extent of the depression of the plasma cortisol is some indication of
the potential for serious PA axis suppression in longer-term clinical
use.

Some investigators have studied the plasma cortisols of patients
being treated with topical corticosteroids and have suggested that
these are more useful in evaluation of PA axis suppressive capacity[14].
The values derived are certainly significant for the group of patients
investigated, but the predictive capacity of this type of observation is
very limited as at present it is not possible to quantify with any degree
of precision the extent of the dermatoses of the particular group of
patients or the degree of barrier defect that is present in them. One
point is clear, however: in PA axis suppression tests, measurement of
plasma cortisol is sufficient. There is no point in trying to 'gild the lily'
and measure urinary metabolites or perform 'adrenal cortex
stimulation' tests in addition. These other tests give little further
information.

Skin thinning action of corticosteroids

The association of striae distensae with spontaneously occurring
Cushing's syndrome and with orally administered corticosteroid
drugs had established that the corticosteroids had a damaging effect
on dermal connective tissue many years ago. However, it was not
until the early and mid-1960s that it came to be generally realized that
topically administered corticosteroids could have a similar effect.
Clinical signs of this action of corticosteroids include the appearance
of skin atrophy and increased fragility of the skin, striae distensae
(especially around major flexures) ecchymoses, and reddening of
facial skin (also due to skin thinning). It is uncertain how this effect on
the dermis is mediated. It has been proposed that corticosteroids are
antimitotic for fibroblasts[15], that they inhibit fibroblast synthesis of
collagen and glycosaminoglycans[16], and that they induce the release
of collagenase[17]. Epidermal thinning is also seen after use of topical
corticosteroids[18]; however, it is unlikely that this contributes sub-
stantially to the clinical appearance noted.

Whatever the mechanisms involved, it has become important to
characterize the 'atrophogenic' effect of new corticosteroid products
and compare this with that of existing materials. It should be noted

that it is more accurate to talk about skin thinning rather than atrophy in the various tests devised, as skin thinning is what is actually measured.

Studies conducted *in vitro* (e.g. Ref. 16) may provide interesting information with regard to biochemical mechanisms. However, they are not likely to be useful in predicting the dermal thinning potential of a particular preparation because the vehicle of the finished product may well influence the degree of skin thinning produced. Neither are *in vivo* animal experiments of much help[19] as small mammals seem to metabolize the various corticosteroid molecules differently[20]. It appears that the most useful types of test are those conducted in healthy human volunteer subjects. Nonetheless there are limitations to even this type of test as there will be differences in the percutaneous penetration between normal individuals' skin and the skin of patients with corticosteroid-treated dermatoses. Furthermore it becomes impractical to ask volunteers to comply with applications for more than 4 or at the most 6 weeks. Clearly the thinning that is produced in this short time is unlikely to be due to loss of collagenous connective tissue alone, as this tissue has a half-life of 6–9 months and inhibition of synthesis of new collagen is unlikely to be evident at 4 weeks. In fact our studies show that with the potent steroids, significant thinning is evident in a few days[21]. This degree of rapidity suggests that movements of tissue fluid may be involved in skin thinning – possibly as a result of the degree of polymerization of connective tissue proteoglycan.

We have found that the most convenient, least invasive, and most reproducible technique for measurement of dermal thickness after the application of corticosteroids experimentally is to use ultrasound[21,22]. The ultrasound device employed (Cutech Ltd) is specially designed to take measurements from skin as it has a resolution of about $50 \mu m$ (Figure 2; Table 2). An X-ray technique (employing Xerox paper) has also been used[23] and found quite reliable (Figure 3), but is limited to investigation of the forearms and also in the number of observations that can be made (Table 3). Calipers can also detect thinning of the skin[24,25] but the technique is intrinsically less accurate (Figure 4). Frosch has also used the stereomicroscopic appearance of the skin surface to detect skin thinning due to application of corticosteroid preparations[27]. However, the observations require considerable skill and experience in interpretation and the technique suffers from the

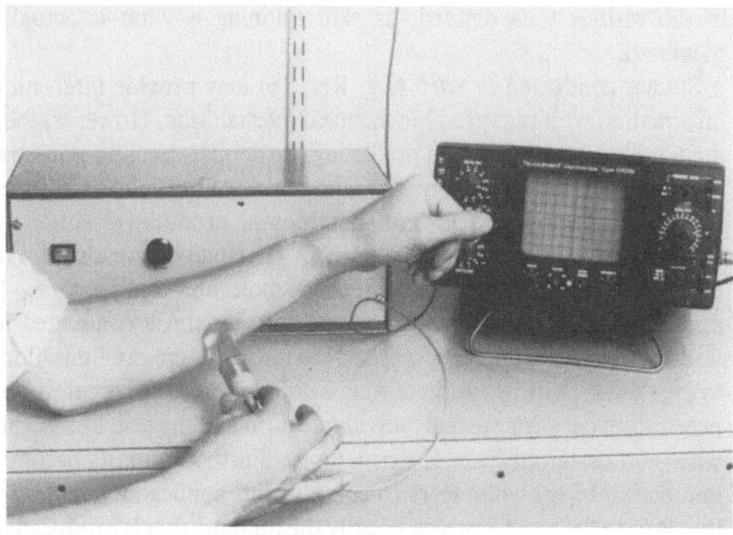

(a)

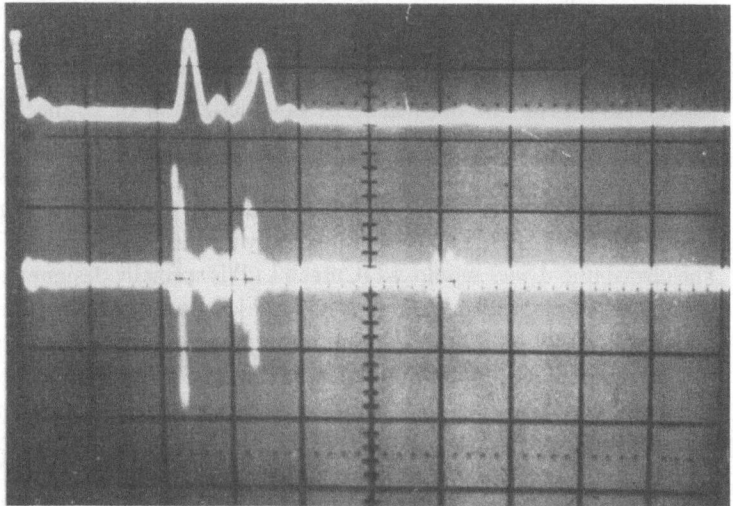

(b)

Figure 2 **(a)** The ultrasound apparatus in use, measuring skin thickness of forearm skin. **(b)** Ultrasound trace.

Table 2 Time course of mean dermal thickness expressed as percentages ± standard deviation of the pretreatment dermal thickness values measured by ultrasound

Treatment	Day 4–5	Day 8–9	Day 28–30	Day 72 (4 weeks after cessation of treatment)
Clobetasol 17-propionate	90 ± 9	88 ± 8	80 ± 10	94 ± 7
Betamethasone 17-valerate	90 ± 6	90 ± 8	86 ± 7	92 ± 6
Hydrocortisone 17-butyrate	90 ± 7	91 ± 8	85 ± 9	91 ± 8
Clobetasol 17-butyrate	93 ± 5	94 ± 6	91 ± 7	96 ± 6
Hydrocortisone	95 ± 7	96 ± 7	90 ± 8	91 ± 9
Base	96 ± 8	96 ± 7	91 ± 8	95 ± 8

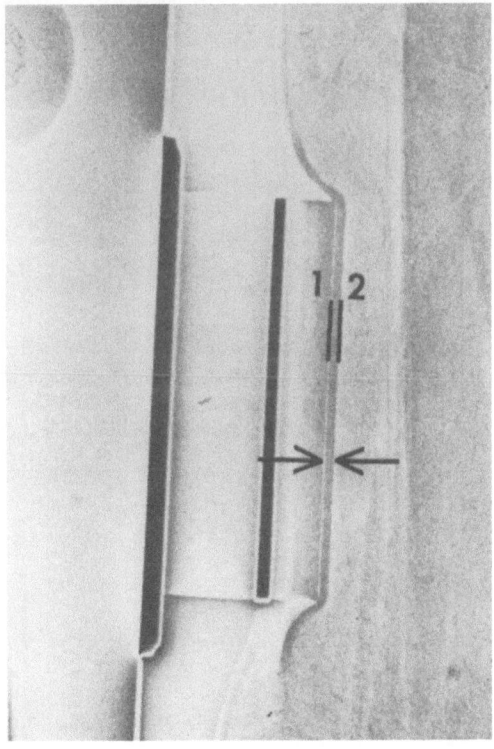

Figure 3 A xeroradiograph of forearm skin taken to measure dermal thickness. The shadow of the dermis is indicated by parallel lines and is measured to obtain the value required

disadvantage of using semiquantitative grading scales. None of the techniques described is perfect but in our view the ultrasound method is the best available at the time of writing.

CONCLUSION

What then is the answer to the question implied in the title? If, despite what has been said, a new corticosteroid preparation is to be taken to the market, then the answer is, as follows, in two parts. Firstly, characterize its properties as completely as possible, and secondly,

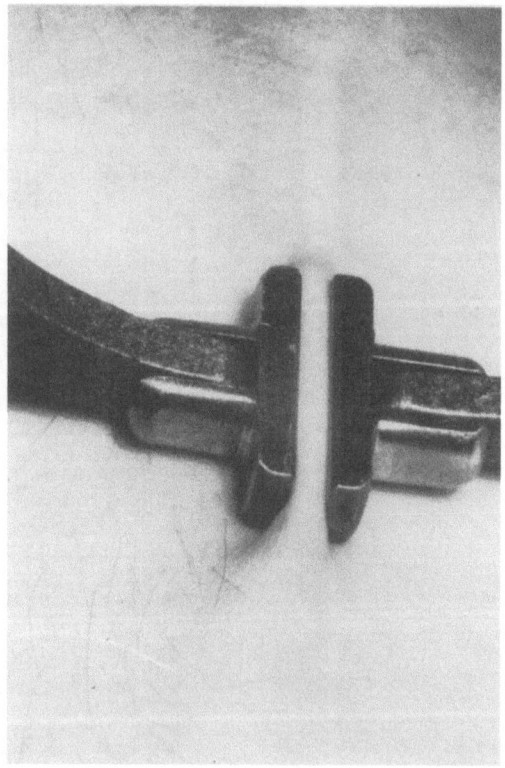

Figure 4   Harpenden calipers being used to measure skin thickness

Table 3 Dermal atrophy after corticosteroid treatment †

Subject	Age	Sex	Dermal thickness* at 4 weeks (mm)		Percentage change
			Placebo	Clobetasol	
1	29	M	1.11	0.95	− 14
2	20	F	0.96	0.74	− 23
3	26	F	0.81	0.73	− 12
4	31	F	0.84	0.58	− 31
5	26	M	1.03	0.76	− 26
6	28	M	1.02	0.76	− 26
7	25	F	0.93	0.87	− 6
8	24	F	0.83	0.76	− 8
9	49	M	1.00	0.94	− 6
Means ± SD			0.95 ± 1.10	0.78 ± 0.12	− 17

*Dermal thickness is expressed as the mean of 6 to 8 readings
†From reference 23

don't let its introduction impede the development and introduction of newer and more interesting compounds.

References

1. McKenzie, A.W. and Stoughton, R.B. (1962). Method for comparing percutaneous absorption of steroids. *Arch. Dermatol.*, **86**, 608
2. Barry, B.W. and Woodford, R. (1974). Comparative bioavailability of proprietary topical corticosteroids preparations: vasoconstrictor assays on thirty creams and gels. *Br. J. Dermatol.*, **91**, 323–338
3. Clanachan, I., Devitt, H.G., Foreman, M.I. and Kelly, I.P. (1980). The human vasoconstrictor assay for topical steroids. *J. Pharmacol. Methods*, **4**, 209
4. Ponec, M., Kempenaar, J.A. and De Kloet, E.R. (1981). Corticoids and cultured human epidermal keratinocytes: specific binding and clinical efficacy. *J. Invest. Dermatol.*, **76**, 211–214
5. Epstein, E.H. and Bonifas, J.M. (1982). Glucocorticoid receptors of normal human epidermis. *J. Invest. Dermatol.*, **78**, 144–146
6. Boxley, J.D., Dawber, R.P.R. and Summerly, R. (1975). Generalized pustular psoriasis on withdrawal of Clobetasol propionate ointment. *Br. Med. J.*, **2**, 225
7. Marks, R. (1982). Effects of emollients on inflammatory dermatoses. In Frost, P. and Horwitz, S.N. (eds.) *Principles of Cosmetics for the Dermatologist.* (St. Louis: C.V. Mosby)
8. Heite, H.U. and Kleinhans, D. (1961). Studie über das quantitativ erfaste Pyrexolerythem bei einigen Dermatosen. *Arch. Klin. Exp. Dermatol.*, **212**, 460

9. Kaidbey, K. H. and Kligman, A. M. (1974). Assay of topical corticosteroids by suppression of experimental inflammation in humans. *J. Invest. Dermatol.*, **63**, 292

10. Kaidbey, K. H. and Kligman, A. M. (1976). Assay of topical corticosteroids. *Arch. Dermatol.*, **112**, 808

11. Marks, R., Pongsehirun, D. and Saylan, T. (1973). A method for the assay of topical corticosteroids. *Br. J. Dermatol.*, **88**, 69

12. Dumas, K. J. and Scholz, J. R. (1972). The psoriasis bioassay for topical corticosteroid activity. *Acta Dermatovener. (Stockh.)*, **52**, 43

13. Gomez, E. L. and Frost, P. (1976). Induction of glycosuria and hyperglycaemia by topical corticosteroid therapy. *Arch. Dermatol.*, **112**, 1559

14. Gomez, E. C., Kaminester, L. H. and Frost, P. (1977). Adrenal effects of new topical steroids. In Frost, P. *et al.* (eds.) *Recent Advances in Dermatopharmacology*. (New Jersey: Spectrum Publications)

15. Berliner, D. L. and Ruhmann, A. G. (1966). Comparison of the growth of fibroblasts under the influence of 11-β-hydroxy and 11-keto corticosteroids. *Endocrinology*, **78**, 373

16. Sarni, H. (1978). Effects of antiinflammatory steroids on DNA glycosaminoglycan and collagen synthesis in vitro. *Thesis*, University of Turku, Finland

17. Houck, J. C., Sharma, V. K., Patel, Y. M. and Gladner, J. A. (1968). Induction of collagenolytic and proteolytic activities by anti-inflammatory drugs in the skin and fibroblasts. *Biochem. Pharmacol.*, **17**, 2081

18. Delforno, C., Holt, P. J. A. and Marks, R. (1978). Corticosteroid effect on epidermal cell size. *Br. J. Dermatol.*, **98**, 619

19. Sim, A. W., Picton, W., Fox, P. K. and Walker, G. B. (1976). The effect of topical corticosteroids on the metabolism of dermal collagen. In Wilson, L. C. and Marks, R. (eds.) *Mechanisms of Topical Corticosteroid Activity*. (Edinburgh: Churchill Livingstone)

20. Young, J. M., Boxall, B. E. and Wagner, B. M. (1978). Topical betamethasone 17-valerate is an anticorticosteroid in the rat. *Br. J. Dermatol.*, **99**, 655

21. Tan, C. Y., Marks, R. and Payne, P. (1981). Comparison of Xeroradiographic and ultrasound detection of corticosteroid induced dermal thinning. *J. Invest. Dermatol.*, **76**, 126

22. Tan, C. Y., Statham, B., Marks, R. and Payne, P. A. (1982). Skin thickness measurement by pulsed ultrasound; its reproducibility, validation and variability. *Br. J. Dermatol.*, **106**, 657

23. Marks, R., Dykes, P. J. and Roberts, E. (1975). The measurement of corticosteroid induced skin atrophy. *Arch. Dermatol. Res.*, **253**, 93

24. Dykes, P. J., Francis, A. J. and Marks, R. (1976). Measurement of dermal thickness with the Harpenden Skin Fold Caliper. *Arch. Dermatol. Res.*, **256**, 261

25. Kirby, J. D. and Munro, D. D. (1976). Steroid induced atrophy in an animal and human model. *Br. J. Dermatol.*, **94** (Suppl. 12), 111

26. Frosch, P. J., Behrenbeck, E. M., Frosch, K. and Macher, E. (1981). The Duhring chamber assay for corticosteroid atrophy. *Br. J. Dermatol.*, **104**, 57

5
Microbial Contamination of Creams

J. R. MORGAN

The quality of pharmaceutical preparations is under considerable threat from a number of factors which may contribute to their deterioration. Not least amongst these is the potential for microbial contamination by bacteria and fungi which, following a period of multiplication, can lead to breakdown of the active ingredient by microbial enzymes or may effect changes in other constituents of the preparation which may in turn combine or alter the active ingredient. At the same time this poses the threat of causing infection in those who use the preparation as with all drugs contaminated during their manufacture. Thus strict aseptic precautions and sterilization techniques must be applied during manufacture to ensure that the product is sterile when first presented to the patient.

With respect to topical preparations there is the added risk of microbial contamination during use which has to be considered. The tube or pot containing the cream or ointment is used repeatedly by the patient over a varying period of time, which may extend to a number of weeks during which the container is opened intermittently for application to the affected skin surface. The topical is then exposed to two sources of contamination. One from the air which allows entry of ubiquitous bacterial and fungal spores from the environment, and secondly the direct entry of organisms from the fingers of the patient which allows access to the usual skin micro-organisms such as *Staphylococcus, Propionibacterium*, members of the family Enterobacteriaceae, and Pseudomonas. The periods in between use may provide opportunity for the multiplication of these organisms within the preparation, particularly if it is stored at room temperature or

61

higher. These problems can be minimized by appropriate education of the patient with respect to the use of sterile applicators to apply the topical to the affected part and instructions to store the cream at domestic refrigerator temperatures in between use. Nonetheless, the risk of contamination is so great as to demand the inclusion in topical preparations of antimicrobial agents which serve to impede the growth of or kill micro-organisms that may contaminate the preparation during its use.

Table 1 lists the features essential to an effective antimicrobial agent. Much is required from such antimicrobial agents, not least of which is the potential to deal with the wide variety of micro-organisms that have the opportunity to gain access. The agent must have a broad antimicrobial spectrum (Table 2), which should include activity against both bacteria and fungi, in particular such fungi as *Candida* spp., *Mucor* and *Aspergillus* and a variety of bacterial pathogens such as *Staph. aureus, Clostridia* spp. Gram-negative organisms such as *E.*

Table 1   Desirable features of an antimicrobial preservative

Broad antimicrobial spectrum:
  Bacteria, spores, fungi, vegetative forms
Bactericidal activity
Non-toxic, potent in low concentrations
Stable
Water-soluble
Non-antagonistic
Non-sensitizing
Non-resistance inducing
Colourless
Odourless

Table 2   Desirable antimicrobial activity of agent

Environmental spores
  Bacillus
  Clostridium
  Fungal

Commensals
  Propionibacterium
  Staphylococcus
  Enterobacteriaceae
  Pseudomonas

coli, Klebsiella and other members of the Enterobacteriaceae, *Pseudomonas aeruginosa,* and beta-haemolytic streptococci. These represent ubiquitous organisms found in dust and as commensals of the human host. The antimicrobial agent must have bactericidal activity. It should actively kill micro-organisms instead of simply preventing them multiplying after contamination of the topical. Whilst it is relatively easy to find compounds that are toxic for bacteria, this toxicity should be selective, that is without toxicity for mammalian cells. This is frequently found to be concentration-dependent; therefore a microbial agent should be potent at lower concentrations, and also stable for long periods of time to coincide with the working shelf-life of the topical.

Bacteria require at least a 15% water content in order to multiply; therefore it is essential that the antimicrobial should be water-soluble, in preference to solubility in the emulsifying agent which would effectively reduce the antimicrobial concentration in the water base of the cream. Since the antimicrobial is present to preserve the efficacy of the active ingredient, it is vital that there should be no antagonistic activity between them. Another important aspect is the capacity of the antimicrobial agent to cause sensitization of the patient and thus result in local or generalized hypersensitivity reaction.

Lastly, there are other factors such as the cost of the agent, its colour, its odour and such other factors which determine its use.

ANTIMICROBIAL ACTIVITY OF PRESERVATIVES

We shall consider only microbial contamination of creams. It is desirable that any antimicrobial agent present should have the capacity to kill pathogens such as *Staph. aureus, Pseudomonas aeruginosa, Salmonella* and *Shigella* spp., *E. coli, Candida* spp. and *Aspergillus* (Table 2). However, it must be borne in mind that almost any microbe has the potential to be pathogenic depending on the clinical circumstances in which it finds itself, particularly in the setting of patients predisposed to infection such as leukaemics and immuno-suppressed individuals. It is an impossible brief to expect an agent to be universally antimicrobial. Nonetheless, there are a number of groups of compounds that have been shown to be potent and useful as preservatives in topical preparations (Table 3). The catalogue is long,

Table 3 Potent antimicrobials suitable for topical preparations

Benzalkonium chloride	Alcohols
Benzyl alcohol	Benzoic acid
Cetrimide	Chloroform
Chlorbutol	Cinnamic acid
Chlorocresol	Formaldehyde
Cresol	Glycerol
Hydroxybenzoates	Sugars
Phenylethyl alcohol	Sulphites
Phenol	
Phenoxyethanol	
Phenylmecurials	

and impossible to discuss in total, but they include the alcohols, phenols, cresols, benzoic acids and derivatives. The first problem encountered is the assessment of the antimicrobial activity of preservatives.

Table 4 illustrates the comparative activity of four compounds measured in aqueous solution against *E. coli*. In terms of time required for sterilization they all are equivalent. However, in terms of residual efficacy after challenge with 10^9 colony-forming units (CFU) of *E. coli*, phenol and m-cresol are superior agents. A vital consideration is the set of conditions under which the antimicrobial agent is expected to have its effect. *In vitro* testing in simple aqueous solution is inadequate other than for screening purposes.

In the real situation, i.e. in the milieu of a topical cream, conditions may interfere with the activity of the antimicrobial. The *British Pharmocopoeia* recommends for the testing of antimicrobial agents that the test be properly performed in the presence of the topical agent. 10^6 CFU of the test organism are mixed in the topical

Table 4 Antibacterial activity of four compounds

Preservative	BP recommended concentrations (%)	Percentage preservative removed by E. coli (%)	Killing time 10^9 E. coli (min)	Residual killing time (min)
Phenol	1.0	0.5	10	10
m-Cresol	0.3	0.6	10	10
Chlorocresol	0.08	2.5	10	11.5
Benzylchlorophenyl	0.006	33	10	115

Derived from Bean (1972)

preparation and also in a water control. Both the tests and the control are sampled at 0 min, 6 h, 24 h, 48 h, 7 days, 14 days and 28 days, and at each time counts of viable micro-organisms are performed. The requirement is that there be a reduction of 10^3 CFU of the test organism within 48 h and a reduction to 0 CFU in 7 days. Bacteriostasis is insufficient; there has to be 'cidal' activity and active reduction in the number of organisms present. However, repeated challenge to assess residual activity is not recommended although in practice the preservative power in a topical is repeatedly challenged.

ANTAGONISM

The relevance of testing the killing activity of an antimicrobial agent in the specific topical agent is the possible antagonistic effect of ingredients within the preparation. A good example of this is documented in an outbreak of *Pseudomonas* infections in a ward in which steroid cream was incriminated. The antimicrobial agent present in the cream was chlorocresol, at a concentration of 0.1%. This was an adequate concentration of chlorocresol since *Ps. aeruginosa* is inhibited by 0.02% of the compound. However, the cream was diluted before use, using a bland cream which contained an accompanying ingredient, 1% cetomacrogol, an emulsifying wax. When the 0.1% of chlorocresol was tested against *Ps. aeruginosa* in the presence of 1% cetomacrogol it was found to be ineffective. This represented a dangerous situation because although *Ps. aeruginosa per se* is not a particularly virulent pathogen, in the context of corticosteroid therapy having a detrimental effect on host resistance, the potential for virulence is enhanced.

When a preservative is included in a topical cream the efficacy of the preservative may be severely impaired due to partitioning of the agent between the oily and aqueous phases of the emulsion and, since bacterial growth tends to take place in the aqueous phase, the consequences are obvious.

Quaternary ammonium compounds, whilst effective in aqueous screening tests as an antimicrobial agent, are frequently found to be ineffective in practice because of loss of activity in the presence of compounds such as lanolin, lecithin, zinc oxide, etc. The parabenz compounds (hydroxybenzoates) are effective agents although somewhat narrow in their spectrum of activity, as they are inactivated in the presence of non-ionic emulsifiers and proteins and furthermore tend to partition in the oil phase of emulsions and so away from the aqueous phase of microbial growth.

Antagonistic potential also exists between the antimicrobial agent and the container. There are many reports in the literature on the subject of the loss of antimicrobial preservatives from rubber cap containers. Although this may seem less relevant in the age of plastics, there are also reports that plastics have a tendency to bind certain antimicrobial preservatives, effectively reducing their antimicrobial availability. Phenylmercuric acetate activity was shown to be diminished by 31% over a 2-week period in contact with polyethylene, and by 12 weeks 66% of the preservative was lost in this way (Table 5).

Table 5 Diminution of antibacterial activity of phenylmercuric acetate in contact with polyethylene

Time (weeks)	Phenylmercuric acetate in plastic (% preservative lost) (RT)
2	31
4	37
12	66

Derived from Lachman (1968)

ALLERGENICITY

The capacity of an antimicrobial agent to produce an allergic response is particularly relevant in the context of topical creams. Assessment of this potential has been explored by means of various human and animal tests. Volunteer studies have shown that while some agents have potent antimicrobial activity they are also potent sensitizers. Bronopol, which is a broad-spectrum antimicrobial agent which includes *Ps. aeruginosa* in its antibacterial spectrum, has been shown to elicit an allergic reaction in 12% of a group of volunteers. Furthermore, of the volunteers shown to be sensitive in this study, a further 20% were found to have become sensitized to formaldehyde. Phenyl mercury compounds, e.g. acetate and chloride, while good anti-microbial agents, have been found to sensitize between 2 and 28% of individuals at concentrations ranging from 0.01% to 0.1%. In contrast, chlorocresol, which is a popular preservative used in cream at 0.2%, appeared to be free of sensitization reactions in 31 volunteers exposed to a 5% concentration of chlorocresol.

In summary the preparation of topical creams with respect to microbial contamination poses two problems. Firstly, manufacturing methods have to minimize all opportunities for microbial contamination and wherever possible to include sterilization steps to eliminate any contamination that does occur. The second problem calls for the inclusion of preservatives which are bactericidal in their effect, wide in their spectrum of activity, stable, cheap and active at a low concentration. Finally, their activity should not be antagonized by other ingredients in the formulation or the nature of the container. While there are a large variety of potential agents available, relatively few of them measure up to these requirements. The assessment of the efficacy of an antimicrobial agent must be performed in the presence of the particular topical agent that is being considered. It must be remembered that once manufactured and found to be safe, topicals should not be tampered with in local pharmacies and that microbial contamination can be further reduced by careful use and adequate storage in between use.

Further reading

Bean, H. S. (1972). Preservatives for pharmaceuticals. *J. Soc. Cosmet. Chem.*, **23**, 703–720

Murray, J. B. and Smith, G. (1968). Current aspects of pharmaceutics: incompatabilities of preservatives. *Pharmacol. J.*, **200**, 87–89

Marzulli, F. and Maibach, H. (1973). Contact sensitization of preservatives. *J. Soc. Cosmet. Chem.*, **24**, 399–421

Rosen, W. and Berke, P. (1973). Modern concepts of cosmetic preservative. *J. Soc. Cosmet. Chem.*, **24**, 663–675

Lachman, L. (1968). Instability of antimicrobial preservatives. *Bull. Parent. Drug Assoc.*, **22**, 127–144

6
Conquering the Skin Barrier

B. W. BARRY

When modern formulators develop dermatological preparations for optimum bioavailability, they may employ two main methods of approach, either singly or combined[1]. The first scheme formulates the vehicle in such a way that the drug has the maximum tendency to leave the base and to partition into the skin, with no intention that the vehicle components should affect the physiochemical properties of the stratum corneum. Thus the vehicle design promotes drug release by simply optimizing the chemical potential (thermodynamic activity) of the medicament. The alternative method of approach is to incorporate into the formulation materials known as penetration enhancers. These are chemicals which themselves permeate the skin, dynamically and reversibly decreasing the resistance of the stratum corneum to the penetration of the drug.

In this paper I want to concentrate on some aspects of our recent work in this field, in which I have had the benefit of working with the following stimulating colleagues and graduate students: Drs D. Southwell and R. Woodford, and A. Akhter, S. Harrison and S. Bennett.

A convenient way in which to subdivide the work is into *in vitro* cadaver skin experiments and *in vivo* investigations using the vaso-constrictor assay.

IN VITRO CADAVER SKIN EXPERIMENTS

Thermodynamic control

The development of topical formulations often requires multiple, lengthy diffusion experiments with limited supplies of human skin. It would be advantageous if we could relate a readily measured physical characteristic of the drug in its vehicle to the extent of percutaneous absorption, with the eventual prospect of predicting and optimizing fluxes without performing any diffusion experiments, or only very few.

Under *ideal* conditions we start with the equation first promulgated by Higuchi[2]:

$$\frac{\mathrm{d}M}{\mathrm{d}t} = \frac{aD}{\gamma h}$$

where $\mathrm{d}M/\mathrm{d}t$ is the flux of drug per unit area through the skin, a is the thermodynamic activity of the drug in its vehicle, D is the diffusion coefficient of the drug in the skin barrier, h is the thickness of the membrane and γ is the effective activity coefficient of the drug in the skin barrier phase. This equation gives the important message that drug flux *should* be directly proportional to the thermodynamic activity in the vehicle, provided that D, γ and h remain unaltered.

To test this hypothesis we used as a model penetrant, benzyl alcohol, dissolved in a variety of simple liquids, i.e. butan-1-ol, butyl acetate, toluene, isopropyl myristate, *n*-heptane, propylene carbonate, and isophorone. We used head space analysis by gas chromatography (GC) to relate the activity of the benzyl alcohol to its molar fraction in each vehicle, taking the GC response to neat benzyl alcohol as unity.

We then used 0.5 mol fraction binary mixtures of benzyl alcohol in the various solvents and determined the benzyl alcohol vapour flux through dermatomed, human abdominal skin using a diffusion cell maintained at 30 °C. The receptor contained 50% aqueous ethanol and samples were analysed by GC.

As predicted by the equation, the steady-state vapour flux values did increase linearly with activity, as found by head space analysis, provided that the solvent did not damage the skin.

An interesting feature of this work was that we found that fluxes from the *liquid* state tended to be higher than those from the vapour, and we are at present investigating this aspect of percutaneous absorption.

Penetration enhancers

For many years, clinical investigators have suggested that substances must exist which could temporarily diminish the impermeability of the skin. Such materials, if they are safe and non-toxic, could be used in dermatology to enhance the penetration rate of drugs and even to treat patients systemically by the dermal route. The most promising candidates appear to increase stratum corneum permeability by reducing the diffusional resistance, by reversibly damaging the layer, or by altering the physicochemical nature of the barrier[1].

As possible penetration enhancers we have investigated compounds such as 2-pyrrolidone, N-methyl-2-pyrrolidone, N-ethyl-2-pyrrolidone, dimethylformamide, Azone, caprolactam, solketal, glycofurol 75, sodium cholate, propylene glycol, oleic acid, oleyl alcohol and diethyl-m-toluamide. In one of our main experimental techniques we tried to mimic the *in vivo* usage of topical drugs by using a

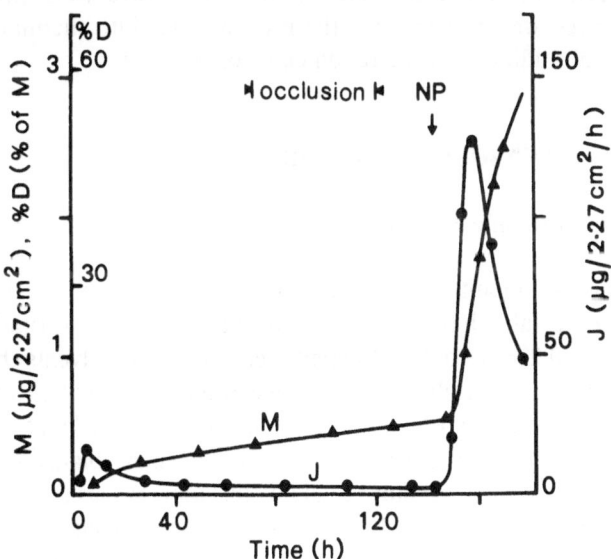

Figure 1 Penetration of ibuprofen through cadaver skin. M represents the cumulative amount penetrated and J is the flux ($\%D$ is the percentage of the dose penetrated). The arrow marks the time at which $100\,\mu l$ of N-methyl-2-pyrrolidone (NP) was added to $700\,\mu g$ of drug deposited from acetone

diffusion cell in which the donor side was open to a controlled temperature and humidity while the receptor phase was kept at 37 °C.

As a typical example of our work in this area, we can consider the results obtained for the penetration of radioactive ibuprofen (a non-steroidal anti-inflammatory agent selected as a model acidic drug). The drug was deposited from acetone as a dry film on dermatomed skin and various treatments were applied. Figure 1 illustrates typical plots of the cumulative amount penetrated (M) and the rate of penetration (J) for a 700 μg deposited film, as a function of time. We see clearly the effect of deposition from acetone, no effect due to occlusion, and a marked effect when 100 μl of N-methyl-2-pyrrolidone was added to the film.

We can turn now to a consideration of some of our results obtained *in vivo*.

The vasoconstrictor assay for topical steroids is an excellent procedure for assessing factors which modify the bioavailability of these drugs by simply scoring the degree of pallor induced on the forearms of volunteers[3]. Just as for the *in vitro* work previously discussed we can subdivide the investigations into thermodynamic control studies and penetration enhancer activity.

IN VIVO VASOCONSTRICTOR (VC) ASSAY

Thermodynamic control

Using our modification of the occluded VC assay we tested six experimental solutions of mechclorisone dibutyrate formulated to contain 0.2% steroid in different blends of polar solvents (hexylene glycol, propylene glycol, propylene carbonate, PEG400, water). All systems were at 90% saturation and therefore *ideally* at the same thermodynamic activity. Figure 2 shows typical blanching curves expressed as the percentage total possible score versus time[4].

From a statistical analysis of our data we concluded that simple thermodynamic control was not operating because the solvent components were not truly inert. For example, such solvents can act as enhancers, irritants, dehydrating agents or they can bind to the drug. Therefore a simpler picture should arise if we only compare similar solvent systems – that is, formulations which use the same

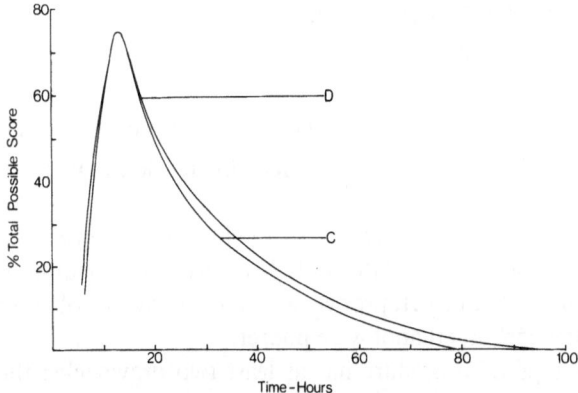

Figure 2 Blanching curves (percentage total possible score versus time) for two 0.2% steroid solutions applied to the arms of 10 volunteers[4]

solvents but in slightly different ratios to maintain constant the thermodynamic activity of the steroid while the overall concentration of the drug may differ. When we investigated this situation experimentally we found that within any solvent system there was no significant difference in the response between preparations containing different concentrations of the steroid but all at 90% saturation. This accords with thermodynamic predictions on the basis that secondary effects (such as penetration enhancement, irritancy, etc.) would be approximately constant within any one solvent system.

We can now turn our attention to the second phase of our *in vivo* studies.

Penetration enhancers

In our first trial we assessed the bioavailability of 0.1% beta-methasone 17-benzoate in a number of solvents which had been suggested as potential penetration enhancers, again using the occluded VC assay. No attempt was made to adjust the steroid concentration to a constant thermodynamic activity, neither was any allowance made for different partition coefficients (stratum corneum to solvent). We were simply looking for dramatic effects[5].

If we take as a standard solution the steroid dissolved in dimethylisosorbide, DMI (*not* an enhancer) then we can determine bio-availabilities from

$$\text{Bioavailability} = \frac{\text{AUC of steroid in test solution}}{\text{AUC of steroid in DMI}}$$

Here AUC stands for 'area under the blanching curve'.

In this study we found that only *N*-methyl-2-pyrrolidone was statistically better than DMI; propylene glycol, diethyl-m-toluamide (Deet) and Deet 75% in ethanol were poorer.

This type of procedure has at least two drawbacks: the lack of thermodynamic control and the *occluded* test procedure. For our second trial therefore we kept the thermodynamic activity of the steroid constant (at 10% saturation) and we tested the systems under *non-occluded* conditions so as to avoid the swamping effect of hydrating the stratum corneum. We used 70% aqueous solutions of

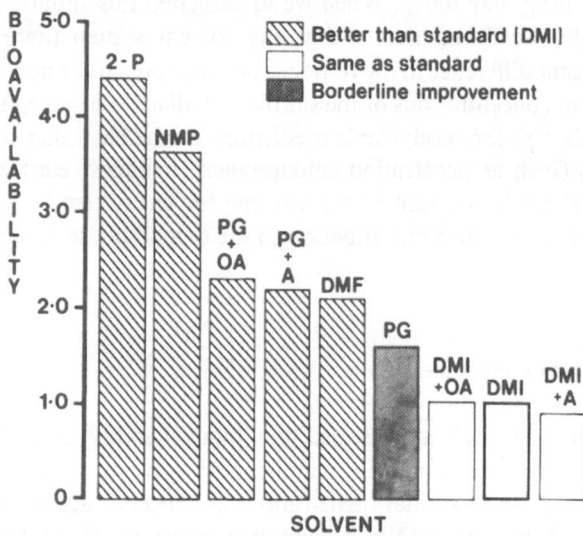

Figure 3 Bioavailabilities for betamethasone 17-benzoate dissolved in various solvents, as assessed by the vasoconstrictor assay (2–P = 2-pyrrolidone, NMP = *N*-methyl-2-pyrrolidone, PG = propylene glycol, OA = oleic acid, A = Azone, DMF = dimethylformamide, DMI = dimethylisosorbide)

accelerants (90% for propylene glycol), approximately 2% Azone and 1.5% or 5% oleic acid. The concentrations of Azone and oleic acid represented saturated solutions of these chemicals, i.e. maximum thermodynamic activities.

Figure 3 represents a histogram of the results which we obtained. Under non-occluded conditions with a standard thermodynamic activity and using DMI as our baseline solvent, we see that 2-pyrrolidone, N-methyl-2-pyrrolidone and propylene glycol plus oleic acid or Azone increased the bioavailability of this steroid. When oleic acid or Azone were incorporated into DMI they did not significantly affect the bioavailability. (For enhancer activity, unsaturated isomers such as oleic acid need to be dissolved in specific polar solvents, such as propylene glycol - Cooper, personal communication.)

The data presented are examples of the work in which we have been involved in Bradford. At present, we are expanding activities in this area and trying to deduce molecular mechanisms to explain many of the data which have been presented in this paper.

Acknowledgement

The author thanks Mrs R. Pyrah for typing this report.

References

1. Barry, B.W. (1983). *Determatological Formulations: Percutaneous Absorption.* (New York and Basel: Dekker)
2. Higuchi, T. (1960). Physical chemical analysis of percutaneous absorption process from creams and ointments. *J. Soc. Cosmet. Chem.,* **11**, 85-97
3. Barry, B.W. and Woodford, R. (1978). Activity and bioavailability of topical steroids. In vivo/in vitro correlations for the vasoconstrictor test. *J. Clin. Pharm.,* **3**, 43-65
4. Woodford, R. and Barry, B.W. (1982). Optimisation of bioavailability of topical steroids: thermodynamic control. *J. Invest. Dermatol.,* **79**, 388-391
5. Barry, B.W., Southwell, D. and Woodford, R. (1984). Optimisation of bioavailability of topical steroids: penetration enhancers under occlusion. *J. Invest. Dermatol.,* **82**, 49-52

7
Release of Drugs from Topical Preparations and their Subsequent Fate

J. HADGRAFT

SUMMARY

The relevance of thermodynamic activity in the formulation of topical preparations is discussed. In some situations the micro-viscosity of the base is also important and the technique of photon-correlation spectroscopy has been used to assess this in some gel systems. The *in vitro* results are compared with some *in vivo* data obtained from a rabbit model. The fate of a topically applied drug may be predicted using a simple pharmacokinetic model which is described.

INTRODUCTION

The overall effectiveness of a topical preparation will depend both on the release characteristics of the base and the subsequent pharmaco-kinetics of the drug as it diffuses through the skin and is removed by the dermal vasculature. The design of the preparation will thus depend on whether the drug is required to act solely at the skin surface or within the layers of the epidermis. Total changes in formulation strategy are required if the topical preparation is to be used as a trans-dermal drug delivery system. In order to optimize the design of formulations it is necessary to understand some of the basic physicochemical principles which influence the release rates of the drugs and their diffusion through the heterogeneous layers that comprise the epidermis.

Some of the factors influencing drug release rates, such as thermo-dynamic activity, microviscosity and particle size, have been assessed in this laboratory and will be discussed. We have also produced mathematical models to predict the effect of partitioning and other simple physicochemical constants on penetration rates. These theoretical descriptions have been combined and simplified into a classical pharmacokinetic model which may be used to predict drug levels in the skin, the plasma and total amounts excreted in the urine. The individual rate constants in the pharmacokinetic analysis can be ascribed to simple physical characteristics of the drug. To date the model has been used to assess the urine excretion data for hydro-cortisone, testosterone and benzoic acid[1].

THERMODYNAMIC ACTIVITY AND VISCOSITY

It has been shown that the chemical potential or thermodynamic activity of drugs in topical bases is an important factor in controlling *in vivo* penetration[2]. Davis and Khanderia[3] indicate that the probable dominant effects in release from topical bases are those of thermo-dynamic activity and viscosity. By considering a simple series of poly-ethylene glycol bases it was possible to show the significance of thermodynamic activity.

In order to assess the thermodynamic activity, head-space analysis by gas chromatography was used. In this procedure the thermo-dynamic activity of a volatile constituent is estimated by allowing a sample to equilibrate in a sealed container. The vapour phase is then analysed by gas chromatography[4].

Methyl salicylate was used as a model drug compound with poly-ethylene glycols as model bases[5,6]. In order to estimate the effects of the thermodynamic activity, the release rates of methyl salicylate from the different PEG bases were measured using a standard diffusion cell[7]. A linear relationship between the amount of drug re-leased and the square root of time was observed as shown in Figure 1. The gradients of the graphs provide an estimate of the apparent diffusion coefficient of the methyl salicylate in the different bases[8,9].

amount released
(μg.ml^{-1})

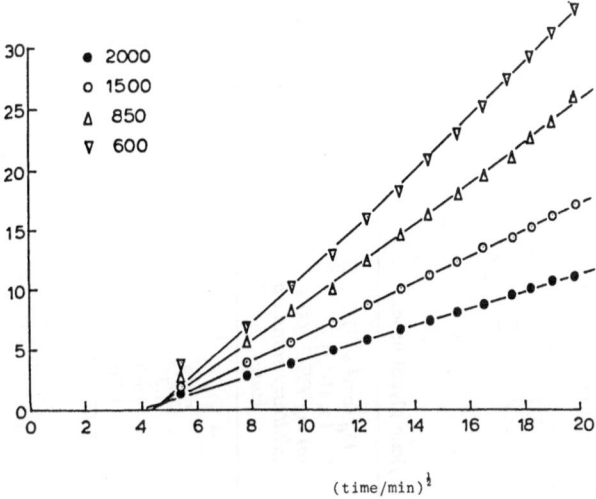

(time/min)$^{\frac{1}{2}}$

Figure 1 The release of 10% w/w methyl salicylate from polyethylene glycol bases at 30 °C. $\triangledown$ PEG 600; $\triangle$ PEG 850 (20% PEG plus 80% PEG 1000); $\circ$ PEG 1500; $\bullet$ PEG 2000

These are summarized in Table 1. The higher the molecular weight of the PEG the lower the diffusion coefficient of the methyl salicylate.

The bases containing methyl salicylate were stored in sealed containers with PTFE caps for 40 days. The concentration of methyl salicylate in the vapour phase was measured and the results presented in Table 1. It is then possible to calculate relative diffusion coefficients (D_R) at constant thermodynamic activity using PEG200 as an arbitrary standard state. The data are presented in Table 1 and show a general fall in D_R with increasing PEG molecular weight, which may be attributed to a viscosity effect.

In vivo absorption of the salicylate from the bases was measured using a rabbit ear model. The base was applied to one ear of a lop rabbit and blood samples collected from the contralateral site. Plasma salicylate concentrations were measured by HPLC. At a given drug concentration the amount of salicylate absorbed was assessed by measuring the area under the plasma level/time curve. The areas are given in Table 1. An excellent *in vitro-in vivo* correlation exists between the values of D_R and the area under the plasma–time curve.

Table 1 Apparent diffusion coefficients 10% w/w methyl salicylate in polyethylene glycol bases

PEG	Effective D (cm² s⁻¹) (×10⁻⁷)	Head space concentration (μg ml⁻¹ × 10⁻²)	D_R (cm² s⁻¹) (×10⁻⁷) taking PEG 200 as arbitrary standard state	Area under plasma level/time curve (mg)
200	–	5.97	–	–
600	1.80	4.11	3.79	1150
850	1.05	3.33	3.37	1000
1500	0.48	2.67	2.40	780
2000	0.20	2.01	1.76	550

Table 2 Apparent diffusion coefficient of polystyrene particles in carbopol 940 gel at different gel concentrations at 30 °C measured by photon correlation spectroscopy and calculated values of microviscosity

Percentage w/w of gel	D cm^2 s^{-1} × 10^{-9}	η cp
0.00	7.87	0.88
0.01	5.20	1.33
0.05	1.38	5.01
0.075	1.18	5.86
0.100	0.87	7.95
0.250	0.72	9.65
0.500	0.51	13.46
0.750	0.42	16.59
1.000	0.34	20.58
1.250	0.28	24.44
1.500	0.23	29.81

This confirms the view that both thermodynamic activity and viscosity are important in determining *in vivo* percutaneous penetration rates.

The importance of viscosity has also been studied using carbopol gels. The microviscosity of a series of carbol 940 gels was estimated by measuring the apparent diffusion coefficient of polystyrene latices of known diameter (0.642 μm) which had been suspended in the gel. The diffusion coefficients were measured using a Malvern Instruments photon correlation spectrometer (PCS). Using the Stokes–Einstein equation the microviscosities of the gel samples at 30 °C were calculated and are given in Table 2.

. Methyl salicylate in the carbopol gels was applied as before to the rabbit ear and area under the plasma–time curve measured. Figure 2 shows that there is a linear relationship between the area under the plasma–time curve and the inverse of the microviscosity of the gel as determined by PCS.

Particle size

The *in vitro* release and *in vivo* absorption of salicylic acid with a range of particle sizes has been measured. The ointment base chosen for this study was Plastibase 50W. The *in vitro* release was studied using the conventional diffusion cell[7] and the amount of drug released

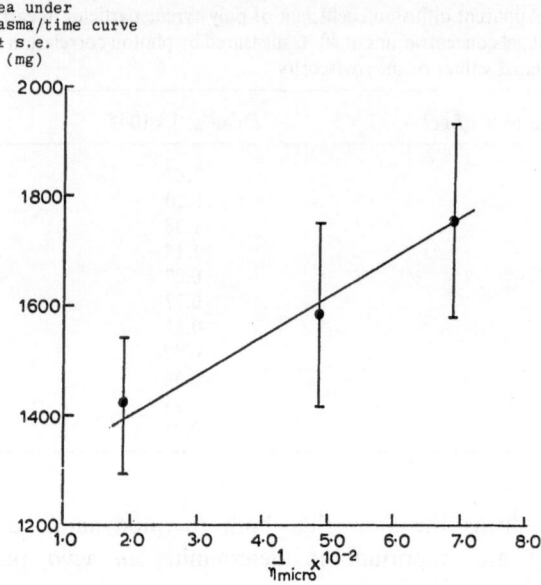

Figure 2 Area under the plasma/time curve plotted against the inverse micro-viscosity of carbopol gels for 8% w/w methyl salicylate

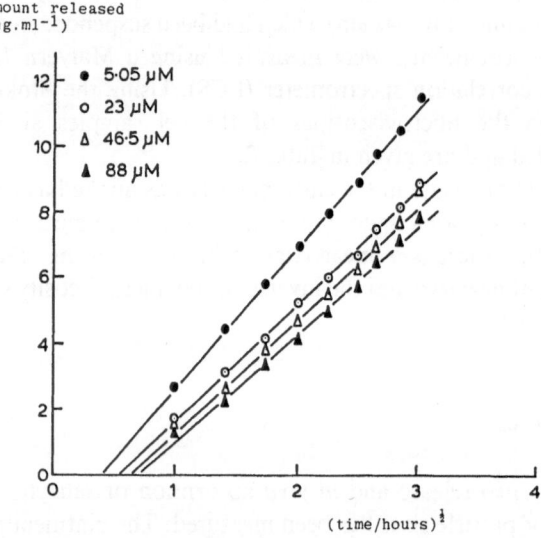

Figure 3 Salicylic acid release (10% w/w) from Plastibase 50W. The results show the effect of the particle size of the incorporated salicylic acid

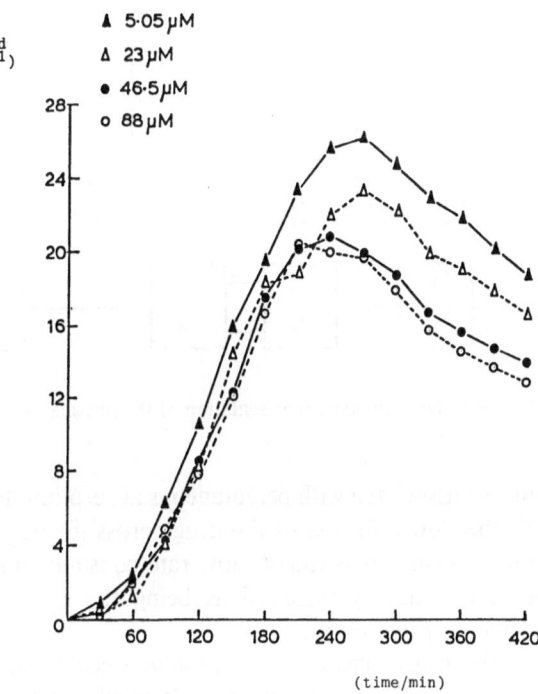

Figure 4 Percutaneous absorption of 10% w/w salicylic acid *in vivo* from Plastibase 50W. The effect of particle size is shown

as a function of the square root of time is given in Figure 3. Good linear relationships are found and the gradients of the lines indicate that as the particle size of the salicylic acid decreases the release rate increases.

Further work was performed with these preparations *in vivo* using the rabbit ear model. The results are shown in Figure 4 and show that, as predicted, there is better drug absorption from the base containing salicylic acid at the smallest particle size.

Pharmacokinetics of percutaneous absorption

A linear pharmacokinetic model containing four first-order rate constants has been constructed[10] and is given in Figure 5. The four rate constants may be ascribed to some of the basic physicochemical

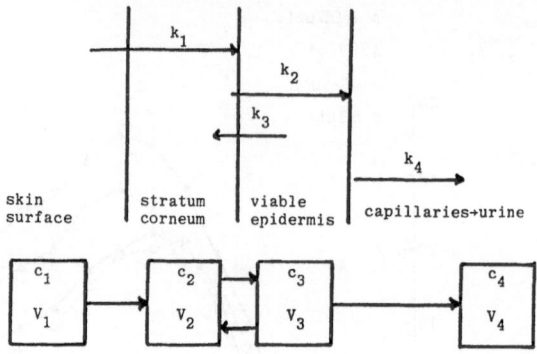

Figure 5 Diagrammatic representation of the pharmacokinetic model

parameters associated with percutaneous absorption. For example k_1 reflects the slow diffusion of the drug across the dead layers of the stratum corneum. It is thus a slow rate constant since the stratum corneum is generally regarded as being the rate-limiting step in percutaneous penetration.

Once the drug arrives at the junction between the stratum corneum and the viable epidermis it encounters a medium which resembles an aqueous protein gel[11]. k_2 may thus be related to the diffusion of drug through an aqueous protein gel medium. Many drugs are known to form reservoirs in the skin by binding to skin components or by simple partitioning phenomena. k_3 reflects the competition for the drug between the primarily lipophilic structure of the stratum corneum and the hydrophilic nature of the viable epidermis. The ratio k_3/k_2 may be understood by considering the 'partition coefficient' of the drug between the stratum corneum and the viable epidermis. Alternatively, the greater the value of k_3, the longer will be the period for which the drug is effectively held up at the stratum corneum–viable epidermis interface.

The fourth rate constant k_4 is effectively the same as the elimination rate constant of the drug following intravenous administration. No attempt has been made to differentiate between drug in the cutaneous capillaries and drug in the general circulation. It was felt that the data available for mathematical analysis are not precise enough to subdivide k_4.

Solution of the first-order kinetic equations is possible using the technique of Laplace transformation[10]. The ratio of the amount of drug that has reached the urine at time t to the amount in compartment 1 at $t=0$, ϕ_t, is given by:

$$\phi_1 = Fk_1k_1k_4 \left[1/k_1\alpha\beta - \frac{e^{-k_l t}}{k_1(k_1-\alpha)(k_1-\beta)} - \frac{e^{-\alpha t}}{\alpha(\alpha-\beta)(\alpha-k_1)} \right.$$

$$\left. - \frac{e^{-\beta t}}{\beta(\beta-k_1)(\beta-\alpha)} \right] \tag{1}$$

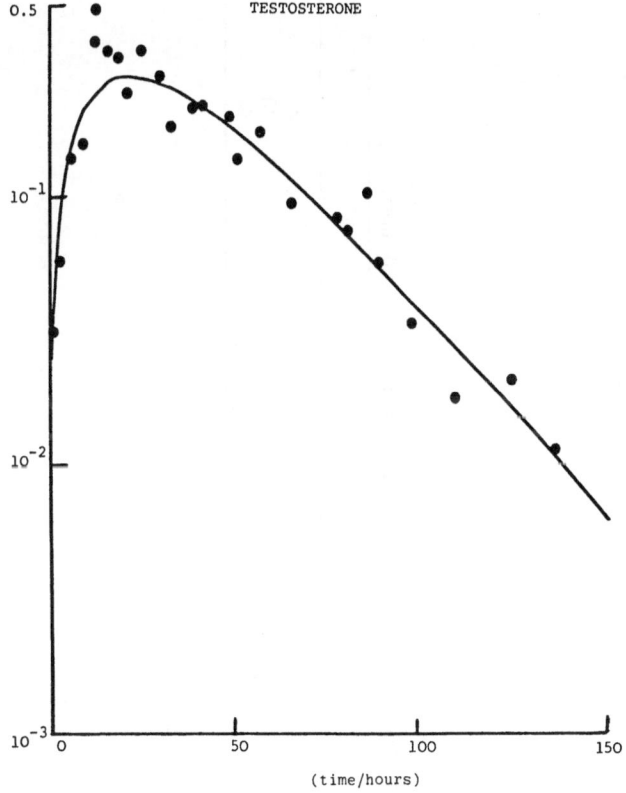

Figure 6 Testosterone: comparison of experimental results (•) and theoretical predictions

Table 3 Physical parameters used to evaluate the theoretical curves

Drug	F^a	$10^5 k_1 \, s^{-1a}$	$10^5 k_2 \, s^{-1b}$	$10^5 k_3 \, s^{-1b}$	$10^5 k_4 \, s^{-1a}$
Testosterone	0.168	1.60	40	75	2.90
Benzoic acid	0.36	5.11	80	0.4	16.45
Hydrocortisone	0.02	0.602	40	5	4.38

a Literature values[1]
b Estimated parameters

where α and β are the roots of the quadratic

$$s^2 + (k_2 + k_3 + k_4)s + k_2 k_4 = 0$$

and F is the fraction of the applied topical dose and metabolites recovered in compartment 4.

Equation (1) was used to analyse urinary excretion data for three compounds; testosterone, benzoic acid and hydrocortisone. The values of the rate constants used are presented in Table 3. Theoretical

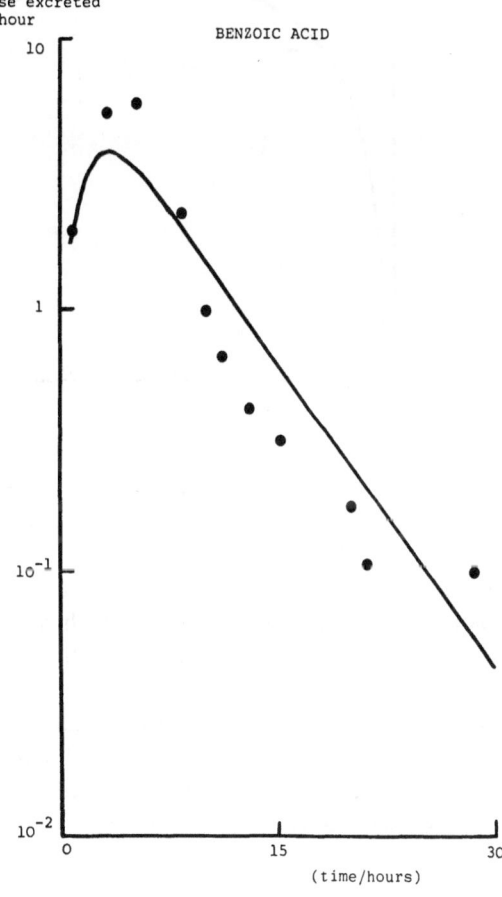

Figure 7 Benzoic acid: comparison of experimental results (•) and theoretical predictions

curves and the experimental data for the three compounds[1] are presented in Figures 6-8. There is good correlation between the theoretical predictions and the experimental points.

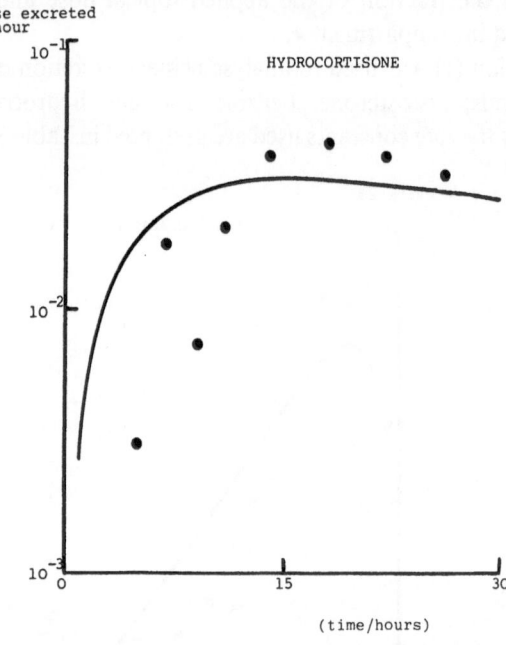

Figure 8 Hydrocortisone: comparison of experimental results (•) and theoretical predictions

The model may be summarized. For drugs cleared rapidly a pharmacokinetic model has been established which may be used to predict urinary excretion data. In order to achieve this, first-order kinetics are used. Good correlation is given between theoretical and experimental results and the rate constants are compatible with physical interpretations and the biophysical conditions. The model is simple yet adaptable enough to prove of general use for the interpretation of percutaneous absorption data.

References

1. Anjo, D. M., Feldman, R. J. and Maibach, H. I. (1980). Methods for predicting percutaneous penetration in man. In Mauvais-Jarvais, P. (ed.), *Percutaneous Penetration of Steroids*. (New York: Academic Press), pp. 31–51.
2. Hadgraft, J., Hadgraft, J. W. and Sarkany, I. (1973). The influence of thermodynamic activity on the percutaneous absorption of methyl nicotinate from water–glycerol mixtures. *J. Pharm. Pharmacol.*, **25**, 122
3. Davis, S. S. and Khanderia, M. S. (1972). Viscoelastic properties of pharmaceutical semi-solids: characterisation of the plastibases for bioavailability studies. *J. Pharm. Pharmacol.*, **24**, 176
4. Achenberg, H. and Schmidt, A. (1977). *Gas Chromatographic Head Space Analysis*. (London: Heyden)
5. Davis, S. S., Hadgraft, J. and Al-Khamis, K. (1981). Percutaneous absorption of methyl salicylate from polyethylene glycol vehicles. *J. Pharm. Pharmacol.*, **33**, 97P
6. Al-Khamis, K., Davis, S. S., Hadgraft, J. and Mills, S. (1982). The determination of thermodynamic activity by gas chromatography head space analysis and its use in studying release rates of drugs from topical preparations. *Int. J. Pharm.*, **10**, 25
7. Billups, N. F. and Patel, N. K. (1979). Experiments in physical pharmacy. V. In vitro release of medicament from ointment bases. *Am. J. Pharm. Educ.*, **34**, 190
8. Higuchi, W. I. (1962). Analysis of data on the medicament release from ointments. *J. Pharm. Sci.*, **51**, 802
9. Hadgraft, J. (1979). Calculations of drug release rates from controlled release devices. The slab. *Int. J. Pharm.*, **2**, 177
10. Guy, R. H., Hadgraft, J. and Maibach, H. I. (1982). A pharmacokinetic model for percutaneous absorption. *Int. J. Pharm.*, **11**, 119
11. Scheuplein, R. J. (1967). Mechanism of percutaneous absorption II. Transient diffusion and the relative importance of various routes of skin penetration. *J. Invest. Dermatol.*, **48**, 79

8
The Clinical Relevance of *in vitro* Investigations for Percutaneous Absorption

B. W. BARRY

When we apply a drug preparation to diseased skin, the clinical response arises from a sequence of three drug-related processes – release of the medicament from the vehicle, followed by its penetration through the skin barriers and finally its activation of the desired pharmacological response. Effective topical therapy optimizes these processes as they are affected by three components – the drug, the vehicle and the skin[1].

Some concept of the complexity of percutaneous absorption may be gained by considering a simple idealization of the drug flux which may arise clinically following the common treatment in which the patient applies a drug to the skin as a solid suspension in a topical vehicle, e.g. an ointment (Figure 1). Drug particles must first dissolve so that their molecules may diffuse within the vehicle to reach the vehicle–stratum corneum interface. Usually interfacial effects are unimportant, but for the drug to move through the skin it must partition into the stratum corneum and then penetrate through this very impermeable barrier. A portion of the drug may bind at a depot site; the remainder diffuses in the horny layer, meets a second interfacial barrier, and partitions into the living epidermis. Although the initial partition process may have favoured an increased flux (for example, when a lipophilic drug is released to the skin from a polar vehicle), the second partitioning will be unfavourable as the living

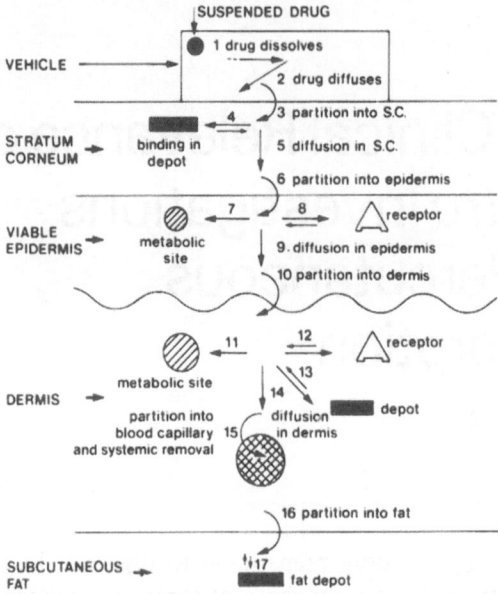

Figure 1 Some stages in percutaneous absorption from a suspension ointment, representing simple unidirectional flux. Emulsion vehicles may also include dissolution and partitioning processes in the internal phase and in micellar pseudophases (Barry[1] – reproduced with permission of the copyright owner)

epidermis provides a more hydrophilic environment compared with that of the stratum corneum. Then a substance with a very low water solubility may not be absorbed percutaneously in active amounts, even though it may have penetrated the barrier layer. The chemical potential of the diffusant in the viable epidermis immediately below the stratum corneum may approach that in the vehicle and in the upper layer of the stratum corneum. The rate-determining step will not now be the penetration of the barrier but rather the clearance from the barrier[2,3]. Metabolism may alter diffusion in the epidermis and it may destroy an active drug or activate a prodrug. We usually assume that the epidermis-to-dermis partition coefficient is near unity as both tissues contain a great deal of water and therefore we neglect it. Within the dermis, additional depot regions and metabolic sites may operate as the drug progresses towards the blood capillary, partitioning into the capillary wall and then out into the blood, from whence the systemic circulation removes it. We know very little about equilibration and pharmacokinetic factors in the subepidermal environment. This knowledge would be particularly important for prodrugs designed for activation in the dermis. Finally, a fraction of the diffusant may partition into the subcutaneous fat or muscle to form a further depot[1].

This sequence of events is too intricate for a full theoretical analysis and a practical investigation. Yet the situation is further complicated. Factors may be important such as the non-homogeneity of the various tissues; the presence of sweat glands, hair follicles, interstitial fluid, and lymphatics; and cell division in the basal layer, their transport through the epidermis and their surface loss. Drugs permeate the skin under dynamic conditions; thus the drug, vehicle components, and the disease process may progressively modify the skin barrier, as may the healing process. Components of the vehicle can diffuse into the skin, and physiological materials, including sweat, sebum and cellular debris, may pass into the formulation and change its physicochemical characteristics. Emulsions may crack or invert when rubbed into the skin and volatile solvents may evaporate into the atmosphere.

When an investigator designs experiments to study this complex

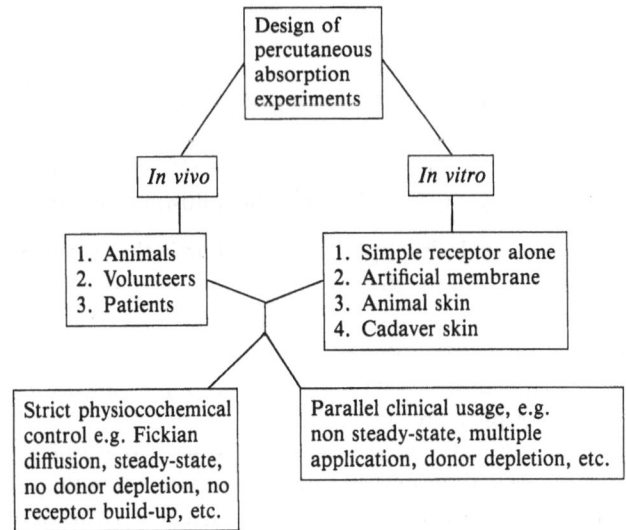

Figure 2   Design of experiments for studying percutaneous absorption

process of percutaneous absorption some of the choices open to him are illustrated in Figure 2. Discussion in this paper will be concerned with the right-hand side of this diagram – the *in vitro* situation. We can identify two main conditions as starting points for our model analysis:

(1) when release from the vehicle provides the rate-limiting step in the process of percutaneous absorption (which means that we ignore the impermeability of the stratum corneum); and

(2) the stratum corneum provides the rate-limiting step for percutaneous absorption (the more usual condition).

We can now examine these two approaches in more detail.

VEHICLE RELEASE IS RATE-LIMITING

Our mathematical treatment assumes that the skin is a perfect sink which maintains essentially zero concentration of the penetrating material by rapidly dissipating it to the deeper tissues. Two general cases worthy of study are absorption from solution and absorption from suspension.

Absorption from solution: skin a perfect sink

We can deduce an equation which relates to the release of a drug from one side of a layer of vehicle under the following conditions[4-6]:

(1) Only a single drug species is important in the vehicle; it is in true solution and the drug is uniformly distributed throughout the vehicle.

(2) Only the drug diffuses from the vehicle. Components other than the drug neither diffuse nor evaporate, and skin secretions do not pass into the vehicle.

(3) The diffusion coefficient of the drug in the vehicle does not change with respect to time or position within the vehicle.

(4) When the penetrant reaches the skin it absorbs instantaneously.

Fickian diffusion theory supplies the simple equation

$$M \simeq 2C_0 \left(\frac{D_v t}{\pi}\right)^{\frac{1}{2}} \qquad (1)$$

M is the quantity of drug released to the sink per unit area of application, C_0 is the initial concentration of solute in the vehicle, D_v is the diffusion coefficient of the drug in the vehicle, and t is the time after application. This equation was originally derived under conditions when the amount of drug released from the vehicle is not much greater than 30%[7], i.e. when t is short[8].

According to the equation, a plot of the amount of drug released as a function of the square root of time should be a straight line. Figure 3 illustrates such a linear relationship for betamethasone 17-benzoate dissolved at various concentrations in a polar gel and diffusing into a chloroform sink[9]. A relationship such as equation (1) or a modification in which the amount of drug released is still proportional to the square root of time will often fit data outside the strict limits used originally to define equation (1), even up to 65% release of drug.

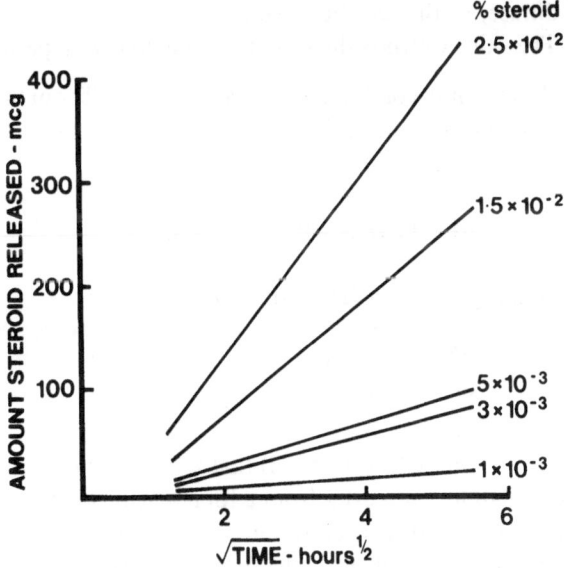

Figure 3 Release of betamethasone 17-benzoate from gel formulations as a function of the square root of time: steroid strength indicated on the plots (Barry[1] – reproduced with permission of the copyright owner)

Absorption from suspensions: skin a perfect sink

The amount released and the rate of release of materials suspended in a topical vehicle may be simply related to time and to the variables of the system; the problem is one of the 'moving boundary' type[4,7]. The relevant model system is described as follows:

(1) The suspended drug is micronized so that the particle diameter is much smaller than the thickness of the applied layer of vehicle.

(2) Particles are uniformly distributed throughout the vehicle and they do not sediment.

(3) The total amount of drug, soluble and suspended, per unit of volume (A) is much greater than C_s, the saturation concentration or solubility of the drug in the vehicle.

(4) The surface to which the vehicle is applied is immiscible with the vehicle; this means that skin secretions do not pass into the vehicle.

(5) Only drug diffuses from the vehicle; vehicle components do not diffuse, neither do they evaporate.

(6) The skin, which is the receptor, functions as a perfect sink.

For the common condition in which drug solubility in the vehicle is very small and A is appreciable (i.e. A is much greater than C_s) we reach the simple equation

$$M \simeq (2AD_vC_st)^{\frac{1}{2}} \tag{2}$$

Differentiating equation (2) produces equation (3)

$$\frac{dM}{dt} \simeq \left(\frac{AD_vC_s}{2t}\right)^{\frac{1}{2}} \tag{3}$$

We see from equations (2) and (3) that a formulator can manipulate the bioavailability of a drug from a topical semi-solid suspension by altering the total drug concentration, the drug solubility in the vehicle, or the diffusion coefficient of the drug in the vehicle. However, the release rate is proportional to the square root of concentration; thus, doubling the concentration of a drug only increases the release rate by about 40%[10].

We can now turn to the more usual situation in which we cannot ignore the impermeability of the stratum corneum; here, the horny layer provides the rate-limiting step in the overall percutaneous absorption process.

Stratum corneum is rate-limiting

Poulsen[11] highlighted the control which the vehicle may have over the diffusional flux of a drug through the skin. He considered several models which were simple compared with *in vivo* conditions but the predictions worked well in clinical practice, particularly with topical steroids used as anti-inflammatory agents. His models assumed the following:

(1) The stratum corneum provides the rate-limiting step in the absorption process.

(2) The skin is a homogeneous intact membrane; shunt routes, such as those provided by the appendages, are not important.

(3) Only a single drug species is important in the vehicle and it dissolves to form an ideal solution. (We can extend our treatment to drug mixtures, provided that each drug behaves ideally and they do not interact.) The penetrant is non-ionic and unaffected by pH changes in the vehicle.

(4) Only drug diffuses from the vehicle. Formulation components do not diffuse, or evaporate, and skin secretions do not dilute the vehicle.

(5) The diffusion coefficient is invariant with time or position within the vehicle or in the horny layer.

(6) The vehicle and the penetrant do not change the diffusion coefficient within the stratum corneum *during* the absorption process.

(7) The penetrant which reaches the viable tissue sweeps immediately into the systemic circulation, so that sink conditions apply below the stratum corneum.

(8) The donor phase does not deplete significantly.

(9) The vehicle does not damage the skin or otherwise alter its permeability *during* an experiment by, e.g. altering the hydration state of the stratum corneum or by functioning as a penetration enhancer.

(10) The drug remains unaltered and intact.
(11) Flux estimates are steady-state values.

Again, we arrive at a very simple equation, the elementary zero order flux diffusion model

$$\frac{dM}{dt} = \frac{KC_vD}{h} \tag{4}$$

Here dM/dt is the steady-state flux of penetrant per unit area of membrane; K is the partition coefficient of the drug between the horny layer and the vehicle; C_v is the concentration of drug *dissolved* in the vehicle; D is the diffusion coefficient of the drug in the stratum corneum; and h is the thickness of the stratum corneum.

When using this equation we usually assume that h is constant and we estimate changes in the penetration rate of the drug from variations in the product KC_vD. Thus the model consists of a vehicle which contains a specified total concentration of drug (dissolved and suspended) in contact with a skin surface of fixed thickness and area.

VIOLATIONS OF THE MODEL APPROACH TO SKIN PERMEATION

In the laboratory we often study simple topical formulations of chemically ideal components applied to membranes which are assumed to be uniform and homogeneous under closely controlled, invariable conditions. However, in therapeutic use, topical formulations are often multiphase, complex and ill-understood, the healthy skin is a diverse, laminated, specialized organ which becomes even more complex in disease, and the conditions under which drugs permeate the skin vary and are not simple. We therefore need to appreciate both the rigorous assumptions employed in model analysis together with how clinical usage violates these suppositions. We can now summarize the main deviations from the ideal conditions which can occur during skin permeation *in vivo*. We will concentrate on the model condition in which we assume that the horny layer provides the rate-limiting step. The set of infringements which we can identify broadly include those which also occur for the vehicle rate-limiting situation.

In general, we have assumed that the horny layer provides the rate-limiting step in the process of percutaneous absorption. However, the patient's skin may become permeable because of disease or damage. The vehicle may occlude the tissue, raising its moisture content and temperature, and thereby decreasing its resistance and its rate-determining role. In clinical use, following application to the skin, the vehicle may change so as to reduce drug diffusion and release from the applied layer. Such alterations may tend towards vehicle control permeation.

The skin is not a simple homogeneous intact membrane but consists of a laminated structure pierced by appendages. These appendages may provide shunt routes for the penetration of electrolytes, large polar molecules and possibly many dermatological drugs[12-14].

Drugs are often not ideal, they may be ionic, and they may be affected by the initial pH of the vehicle and the way in which the pH changes after the vehicle has been applied to the skin.

Seldom is a single drug the only diffusing species. Other drugs may diffuse and affect the permeation of the primary agent. Similarly, low molecular weight solvents may leave the vehicle and diffuse into the skin.

Model analysis usually assumes that the colloidal structure and composition of any vehicle remains constant after it has been applied to the skin. However, phase changes may occur and other alterations to the formulation may take place as the patient rubs the base into the skin; we know very little about how such changes may affect skin penetration. In practice, vehicle components often evaporate or diffuse out of the vehicle, and skin secretions may well penetrate into the formulation. These processes will alter the physicochemical environment within the cream or ointment, compared to conditions which hold within the container. Concentration changes arising from the loss of volatile components from a vehicle may even be used to promote drug penetration through the skin[15]; such enhancement probably occurs with many creams, gels and lotions.

One of our assumptions is that neither the vehicle nor the penetrant dynamically alter the drug's diffusion coefficient within the barrier phase. However, as permeation proceeds, the pH of the stratum corneum and its hydration state may well alter. The integrity of the barrier may decrease and it may even suffer structural damage. The diffusivity of the drug may then not be independent of the time or position within the barrier, or of drug concentration within the skin.

The living tissues may not function as a perfect sink; very non-polar drugs may be so water-insoluble that only a negligible amount partitions from the horny layer into the epidermis and the flux across the stratum corneum becomes minimal. Thus the stratum corneum may well absorb reasonable quantities of drug but not pass the drug on to the site of action in, e.g. the dermis. The drug may also bind to components of the horny layer or induce vasoconstriction and thereby decrease the efficiency of the dermis as a sink.

Much skin permeation work assumes that the penetrant concentration or activity in the vehicle remains constant during permeation. However, in practice this assumption may often not hold. Thus, finite amounts of drug may leave the vehicle and enter the skin; the skin may absorb vehicle components or dilute the preparation with tissue fluids, with resulting effects on the thermodynamic activity of the drug. The drug may precipitate or supersaturate the vehicle as solvents leave; emulsions may invert, and pH changes may affect ionic drugs.

We often assume that the vehicle is inert with respect to any effect it may have on the state of the skin. However, occlusive vehicles hydrate the skin and high concentrations of, for example, glycols, may dehydrate the horny layer. Many low molecular weight vehicle components such as propylene glycol pass rapidly into the stratum corneum and once there they may increase the solubility of the drug in the layer of the stratum corneum in which the vehicle component concentrates.

It is often assumed that the drug remains intact during permeation. However, the drug may be chemically degraded by, e.g. hydrolysis, photolytic action, or metabolism. The vehicle or skin may complex or sorb the drug.

In a typical *in vitro* experiment, flux estimates are usually assumed to be steady-state values. In the clinic such conditions may never be achieved as material is lost from the skin, dermatologicals are reapplied several times daily, and the microenvironment of the skin changes dynamically.

From considerations such as those detailed above we conclude that we need an increased effort devoted to skin investigations under conditions which more closely reflect clinical circumstances[1,16]. We need to link more closely two main streams of investigation, which we can designate as the physicochemical approach (as detailed here) and the biological approach which mimics clinical usage of drugs. We need a synthesis of both outlooks for a successful attack on a dermatological problem which is to be approached via topical therapy.

Acknowledgement

The author thanks Mrs R. Pyrah for typing this report.

References

1. Barry, B.W. (1983). *Dermatological Formulations: Percutaneous Absorption*. (New York and Basel: Dekker)
2. Higuchi, T. (1977). Prodrug, molecular structure and percutaneous delivery. In Roche, B. (ed.), *Design of Biopharmaceutical Properties Through Prodrugs and Analogs*. (Washington, DC: American Pharmaceutical Association), pp. 409–421
3. Higuchi, T. (1978). Design of chemical structure for optimal dermal delivery. *Curr. Probl. Dermatol.*, **7**, 121–131
4. Higuchi, T. (1960). Physical chemical analysis of percutaneous absorption process from creams and ointments. *J. Soc. Cosmetic Chem.*, **11**, 85–97
5. Higuchi, W.I. (1961). Diffusion in ointment bases. *Proc. Am. Soc. Coll. Pharm., Teachers Seminar.*, **13**, 162–173
6. Higuchi, W.I. (1962). Analysis of data on the medicament release from ointments. *J. Pharm. Sci.*, **51**, 802–804
7. Higuchi, T. (1961). Rate of release of medicaments from ointment bases containing drugs in suspension. *J. Pharm. Sci.*, **50**, 874–875
8. Malone, T., Haleblian, J.K., Poulsen, B.J. and Burdick, K.II. (1974). Development and evaluation of ointment and cream vehicles for a new topical steroid, fluclorolone acetonide. *Br. J. Dermatol.*, **90**, 187–195
9. Barry, B.W. and Woodford, R. (1978). Activity and bioavailability of topical steroids. *In vivo/in vitro* correlations for the vasoconstrictor test. *J. Clin. Pharm.*, **3**, 43–65
10. Katz, M. and Poulsen, B.J. (1971). Absorption of drugs through the skin. In Brodie, B.B. and Gillette, J. (eds.), *Concepts in Biochemical Pharmacology*. (Berlin, Heidelberg, New York: Springer) (*Handbook of Experimental Pharmacology*, vol. 28, pt. 1, pp. 103–174)
11. Poulsen, B.J. (1972). Diffusion of drugs from topical vehicles: an analysis of vehicle effects. In Montagna, W., Van Scott, E.J. and Stoughton, R.B. (eds.), *Pharmacology and the Skin*. (New York: Appleton-Century-Crofts) (*Advances in Biology of Skin*, vol. 12, pp. 495–509)
12. Scheuplein, R. J. (1978a). The skin as a barrier, skin permeation, site variations in diffusion and permeability. In Jarrett, A. (ed.), *The Physiology and Pathophysiology of the Skin*. (London, New York, San Francisco: Academic Press), vol. 5, pp. 1669–1692, 1693–1730, 1731–1752

13. Scheuplein, R. J. (1978b). Permeability of the skin: a review of major concepts. *Curr. Probl. Dermatol.*, **7**, 172–186
14. Scheuplein, R. J. and Blank, I. H. (1971). Permeability of the skin. *Physiol. Rev.*, **51**, 702–747
15. Coldman, M. F., Poulsen, B. J. and Higuchi, T. (1969). Enhancement of percutaneous absorption by the use of volatile : nonvolatile systems as vehicles. *J. Pharm. Sci.*, **58**, 1098–1102
16. Franz, T. J. (1978). The finite dose technique as a valid *in vitro* model for the study of percutaneous absorption in man. *Curr. Probl. Dermatol.*, **7**, 58–68

9
The Permeability of Abnormal Skin

R. C. SCOTT

Although the skin has been classically regarded as an almost absolute barrier to the entry and exit of chemicals, scientists have been studying its permeability for many years. Mussey[1] and Reilly[2] published some of the earliest (modern times) demonstrations of skin permeability. By 1929 Schwenkenbecker[3] had demonstrated the preferential absorption of lipophilic molecules, thus stimulating the study of factors governing percutaneous absorption. That sufficient chemicals can be percutaneously absorbed to elicit systemic effects has been proven[4] and fatal amounts of phenol unfortunately witnessed[5]. The known permeability of the skin has made possible its use as a deliberate route of entry for corticosteroids[6] and other drugs such as scopalamine[7]. Of course, the movement of chemicals is not unidirectional and chemicals such as salts and water[8] pass from the body to the atmosphere.

The above studies concentrated on normal, healthy skin with an intact stratum corneum. The stratum corneum is usually the rate-limiting barrier for the entry and exit of most chemicals[9]. Skin covered by an abnormal stratum corneum has been shown to be more permeable than normal skin[10-12]. The reader will be able to compile a list such as Table 1 by scanning the available literature. The table shows a range of chemicals reported to be more readily absorbed through a variety of abnormal skins. However, the absorption of all chemicals is apparently not enhanced through abnormal skin (Table 2).

Studies of absorption through abnormal skin have usually been made at a specific time point. Any permeability changes which may

Table 1 Examples of chemicals reported to penetrate damaged skin more readily than normal skin

Chemical	Species	Damage
n-butanol	hairless mouse	heat
Cobalt	guinea pig	strip
Desoxymethasone	man	strip
Essential fatty acids	rat	strip
Hydrocortisone	man	strip
Galacturonic acid	man	strip
Ions	man	chemical
Methotrexate	man	strip
Nandrolone decanoate	man	strip
Nicotinic acid	man	heat separation
Pyridinethione	monkey	abrasion
Salicylic acid	guinea pig	strip
Sarin	man	strip
Sodium	rat	chemical
Testosterone	man	strip
Triamcinolone acetonide	man	psoriasis

Table 2 Examples of chemicals reported to have no greater absorption through damaged skin compared with normal skin

Chemical	Species	Damage
Clioquinal	man	dermatitis
Diflorasone diacetate	rat, monkey	abrasion

have occurred during epidermal repair/regeneration have not been measured. Such changes do occur and have been measured, though only for a few chemicals such as water and ions[10,13]. These studies show that the permeability of abnormal skin can change hourly. Established, non-invasive techniques are available which permit the permeability of abnormal skin to be measured simply and quickly. Unfortunately, these methods usually measure only water permeability (transepidermal water loss, TEWL) and this cannot be regarded as a reliable guide to the permeability of the skin to other types of chemicals[14]. However, the permeability of many abnormal skin conditions can be 'graded' to indicate the degree of alteration and to follow any repair process. Precisely what these TEWL changes mean for very different molecules, such as drugs which might contact abnormal skin, is presently not known. Several techniques are available for studying and measuring TEWL and these have been well documented[15]. For our studies we used a 'ventilated chamber' technique[14]. During measurements ambient air or a very dry gas such as nitrogen is passed over the skin (Figure 1) and the water content of the gas detected by sensors allowing a calculation of TEWL. Although ambient air is a more physiologically normal medium in which to make the measurement, TEWL through normal intact skin is low and the water sensors must possess a very high degree of resolution to detect any changes in the water content of the gas. The technique has been widely used to study changes in TEWL through human skin after, for example, tape stripping, the application of alkaline liquids[10] and industrial solvents[16]. Similarly, the permeability

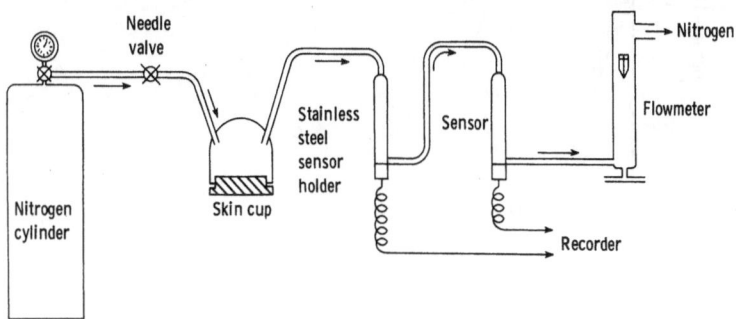

Figure 1 Diagram of the 'ventilated chamber' apparatus used to measure trans-epidermal water loss[20]

of various dermatoses has been measured[17] with psoriatic skin being more permeable (to water) than eczematous or erythrodermatous skin; surprisingly, ichthyotic skin was only slightly more permeable than normal. Using a similar technique, permeability changes were measured in rats with a dietary-induced abnormal skin and the changes during normal barrier production followed after the provision of essential fatty acid[18].

We have studied TEWL changes through rat skin after superficial alterations to the epidermis which removed different proportions of the outermost, dead horny layer, the stratum corneum. The TEWL changes with time, as the permeability barrier regenerated, were

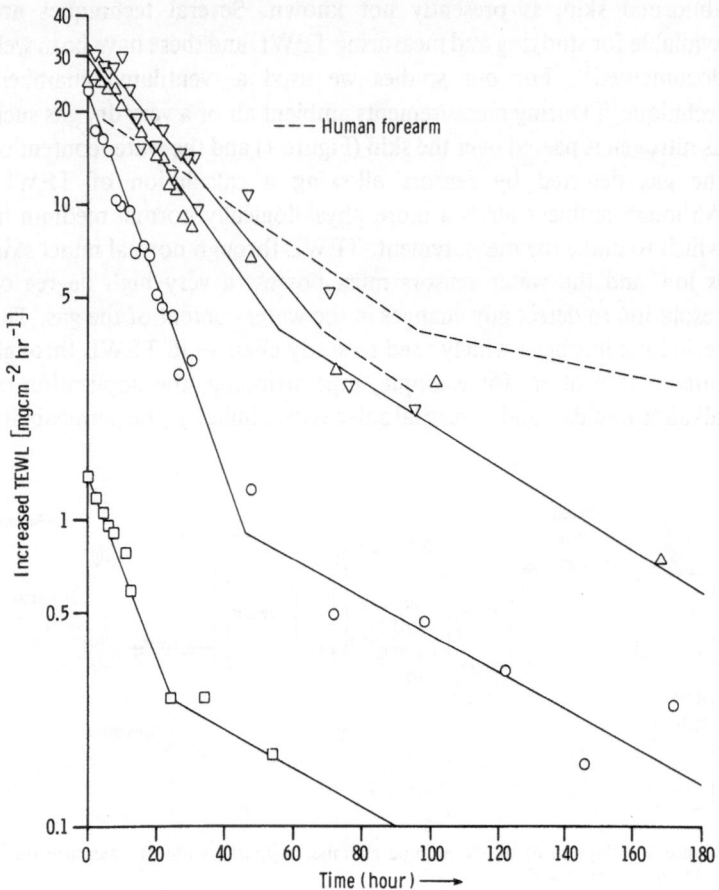

Increased TEWL [mgcm^{-2} hr^{-1}]

--- Human forearm

Time (hour) ⟶

Figure 2 Plot of log permeability (increased transepidermal water loss against time) following four types of mild, superficial alterations of rat skin together with data from similarly treated human forearm skin

measured. These data are summarized in Figure 2 where log increased TEWL is plotted against time. The pattern of permeability changes was similar after each type of alteration: an initial exponential phase accounting for the major portion of barrier regeneration followed by a second, more gradual phase of permeability change, as the permeability returned to normal. The first phase coincided with scab formation over the damaged area and development of a few new layers of stratum corneum. In the second phase the stratum corneum thickened and matured[19]. The dotted line on Figure 2 shows data obtained on human forearm[10] similarly altered as in our study. The TEWL was measured by a similar 'ventilated chamber' technique. The human skin had a similar increase in permeability as occurred in the rat skin and the permeability barrier regenerated in a similar biphasic manner; however, the rat skin regenerated faster than the human.

Physical alteration of the skin leads to an immediate increase in permeability and in the examples we studied maximum TEWL was measured immediately or within hours. However, after some skin treatments changes may occur over a longer time period with maximum permeability measured many hours or days after the insult. We studied permeability changes[20] after a single application of n-hexadecane to rat skin; n-hexadecane is known to affect epidermal differentiation. Together with our 'ventilated chamber' apparatus we also used a Servomed Evaporimeter to measure TEWL. In the evaporimeter the measuring head is open and contains two sensors which measure water diffusing across them and computes the TEWL. The instrument is easy to use and measures under ambient conditions. Both techniques (Figure 3) measured increased skin permeability 5 h

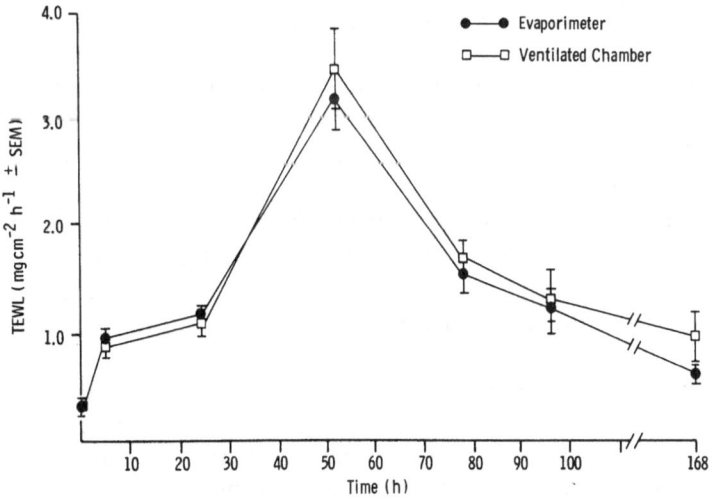

Figure 3 Transepidermal water loss through rat skin treated with a single dose of n-hexadecane, measured on a 'ventilated chamber' system and an Evaporimeter

after application of the *n*-hexadecane and showed maximum peak permeability at about 52 h. After this time there was a gradual return to normal. Both techniques similarly quantified the changes in the range of TEWL which occurred.

The Evaporimeter has been shown[21] to underestimate the larger increases in permeability that occur after physical damage. However, the TEWL through skin afflicted with the common dermatoses[17] is well below that measured through physically damaged skin and comparable to that seen in our *n*-hexadecane-treated skin. The Evaporimeter might be very useful for studying barrier repair following different treatments for dermatoses and in the development of new topical products.

Changes in ion mobility (conductance) have also been studied non-invasively through damaged and regenerating skin[13]. Damaged skin has a greater permeability to ions, i.e. higher conductance, than normal skin. Measurements of TEWL and conductance have shown increases in both, as human skin is progressively tape stripped[8]. We studied ion conductance through rat skin altered as described above. Typically, the conductance was increased after insult and became progressively higher before returning to normal, a different profile of permeability changes from that defined by TEWL (Figure 4).

Our results on physically altered skin and those obtained on psoriatic skin[11] show that the permeability to one type of molecule (water) can be increased whilst the permeability to another (ions) is quite normal through the same area of skin. The permeability properties and factors affecting the absorption of chemicals across abnormal skin are not well understood; generalizations are difficult to make confidently.

The similarity of the water permeability barrier changes measured in human and rat skin stimulated the design of an *in vivo* 'model' to be used to quantify absorption through abnormal skin and the factors governing the rate. Our chosen 'model' design is rat skin, stratum corneum removed by tape stripping and allowed to regenerate for 0, 24 (on the first phase of barrier regeneration) and 96 h (second phase). Chemicals were applied to the different 'skin types' (times) and the rate of absorption quantified and compared with normal. Other workers have designed different 'abnormal skin' models (e.g. Solomon and Lowe[22]). We believe our 'model' is particularly useful as the stratum corneum is removed at a precise time. This permits the quantitation at a time (0 h) of maximum barrier disturbance and permeability (as indicated by TEWL) facilitating 'worst case' risk assessment for a chemical contacting abnormal skin. Changes in permeability are measured as the barrier regenerates and these may possibly be related to other hyperplastic skin conditions. Chemical absorption is determined by analysis of an appropriate body fluid.

The percutaneous absorption of a number of chemicals has been studied using the 'model' and its usefulness can be demonstrated by data obtained with [3H]-mannitol. Absorption through the different 'skin types' was quantified by analysis of urine for [3H] and the results are summarized in Table 3. The table shows the percentage of the applied topical dose which accumulated in the urine over 24 h (part B). As the same dose was applied each time, a factor of difference in absorption compared to normal skin can be calculated. In contrast to water (TEWL measurements) no barrier to [3H]-mannitol had formed by 24 h but a barrier had formed by 96 h. The factors of difference quantify the large increases in permeability through the abnormal skin. Chemicals do not, normally, contact skin for 24 h; if

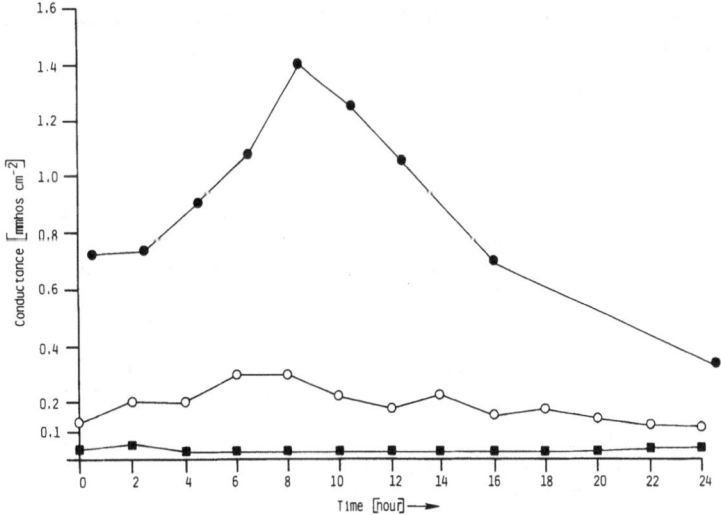

Figure 4 Plot of changes in conductance against time through rat skin following mild superficial alteration, compared to changes through normal skin over the same time period

they are accidentally applied they would be washed off and if, perhaps, a prescribed topical drug, applied more frequently. The 'model' can be used to quantify absorption during variable periods of skin contact (Table 3 part B). We hope this 'model' will be used to aid

Table 3 Mannitol in urine following application to abnormal rat skin

Skin state	Percentage of topical dose excreted and (factor above normal)	
	A	B
	3 h after application	24 h after application
Normal	0.07	0.42
0 h Recovery	34 (420)	52 (140)
24 h Recovery	31 (400)	50 (130)
96 h Recovery	0.36 (4)	1.8 (4)

the development of safer, more effective formulations of topical drugs and to study the factors governing the rate of absorption through damaged skin.

Our knowledge and understanding of absorption through normal intact skin is well documented; studies on abnormal skin are in their infancy.

References

1. Mussey, R. D. (1899). Experiments and observations on cutaneous absorption. *Philadelphia Med. Phys.*, **3**, 288–293
2. Reilly, T. F. (1901). The unbroken skin as an absorbing medium. *J. Am. Med. Assoc.*, **56**, 250–253
3. Schwenkenbecker, A. (1929). Die haut ab exkretionsorgan. *Bethe. Handt d. norm u. path Physiol.* (Berlin: Springer), vol. 4, pp. 709–768
4. Abrams, H. K., Hamblin, D. O. and Marchand, J. F. (1950). Pharmacology and toxicology of certain organic phosphorous insecticides. *J. Am. Med. Assoc.*, **144**, 107–108
5. Gottlieb, J. and Storey, E. (1936). Death due to phenol absorption through unbroken skin. *J. Maine Med. Assoc.*, **110**, 409–412
6. Mattila, R. (1980). Betamethasone diproprionate with salicylic acid flumethasone privalate with salicylic acid in steroid responsive dermatoses demanding keratolytic penetration. *J. Int. Med. Res.*, **8**, 247–250
7. Shaw, J. E. and Chandrasekaran, S. K. (1978). Controlled topical delivery of drugs for systemic action

8. Grice, K., Sattar, H., Casey, T. and Baker, H. (1975). An evaluation of Na^+, Cl^- and pH ion-specific electrodes in the study of the electrolyte contents of epidermal transudate and sweat. *Br. J. Dermatol.*, **92**, 511–518

9. Scheuplein, R. J. and Blank, I. H. (1971). Permeability of the skin. *Physiol. Rev.*, **51**, 702–747

10. Spruit, D. (1969). The measurement of the regeneration of the water vapour loss of human skin. *PhD thesis*. Catholic University of Nijmegen, Netherlands

11. Grice, K. A., Sattar, H. and Baker, H. (1973). The cutaneous barrier to salts and water in psoriasis and in normal skin. *Br. J. Dermatol.*, **88**, 459–463

12. Prottey, C., Hartrop, P. J., Black, J. G. and McCormack, J. I. (1976). The repair of impaired epidermal barrier function in rats by the cutaneous application of linoleic acid. *Br. J. Dermatol.*, **94**, 13–21

13. Malten, K. E. and Thiele, F. A. J. (1973). Evaluation of skin damage. II: Water loss and carbon dioxide measurements related to skin resistance measurements. *Br. J. Dermatol.*, **89**, 565–569

14. Scott, R. C. (1982). The permeability of normal and abnormal rat skin. *PhD thesis*. University of Bradford, UK

15. Nilsson, G. E. and Oberg, P. A. (1979). Measurement of evaporative water loss: methods and clinical applications. In Rolfe, P. (ed.), *Non-invasive Physiological Measurements*. (City: Publisher), vol. 1, pp. 279–312

16. Spruit, D., Malten, K. E. and Lipmann, E. W. R. (1970). Horny layer injury by solvents II. Can the irritancy of petroleum ether be diminished by pretreatment? *Berufsdermatosen*, **18**, 296

17. Grice, K. A. and Bettley, F. (1967). Skin water loss and accidental hypothermia in psoriasis, ichthyosis and erythroderma. *Br. Med. J.*, **4**, 195–198

18. Hartrop, P. J. and Prottey, C. (1976). Changes in transepidermal water loss and the composition of epidermal lecithin after applications of pure fatty acid triglycerides to the skin of essential fatty acid-deficient rats. *Br. J. Dermatol.*, **95**, 255–264

19. Scott, R. C., Dugard, P. H. and Doss, A. W. (1985). The permeability of abnormal rat skin. *J. Invest. Dermatol.* (To be published)

20. Scott, R. C., Oliver, G. J. A. O., Dugard, P. H. and Singh, H. J. (1982). A comparison of techniques for the measurement of transepidermal water loss. *Arch. Dermatol. Res.*, **274**, 57–64

21. Wheldon, A. E. and Monteith, J. L. (1980). Performance of a skin evaporimeter. *Med. Biol. Eng. Comput.*, **18**, 201–208

22. Solomon, A. E. and Lowe, N. J. (1978). Percutaneous absorption in experimental epidermal proliferation. *Arch. Dermatol.*, **114**, 1029–1030

10
Topical and Oral Preparations of Glyceryl Trinitrate – A Comparative Study

M. J. LEWIS, A. BASHIR and A. H. HENDERSON

Organic nitrates such as glyceryl trinitrate (GTN) are available in several different dosage forms, e.g. sublingual, oral and topical. The requirement for so many pharmaceutical preparations stems mainly from the short-lived pharmacological effect of these compounds and the resultant attempts to prolong it.

The major pharmacological action of all organic nitrates including GTN is to relax smooth muscle. This effect is mediated by the intracellular generation of inorganic nitrite ions (NO_2^-)[1,2] which can efflux from the smooth muscle cell into the plasma. These inorganic NO_2^- ions are eventually oxidized to inorganic nitrate (NO_3^-) by the liver and kidney[3]. Inorganic NO_2^- (and hence NO_3^-) is also formed from the hepatic breakdown of GTN. Thus plasma levels of these inorganic ions provide some measure of the metabolism of GTN both by smooth muscle and liver. Previous pharmacokinetic studies of GTN have not included measurement of these ions. Accordingly we have measured plasma levels of NO_2^- and NO_3^- together with GTN itself in healthy male volunteers who were given single doses of five different pharmaceutical preparations of GTN. The plasma measurements were made with newly developed gas–liquid-chromatographic techniques validated in the usual way.

Six healthy male volunteers (aged 25–32 years) were given single doses of each of the five GTN preparations at intervals of > 1 week.

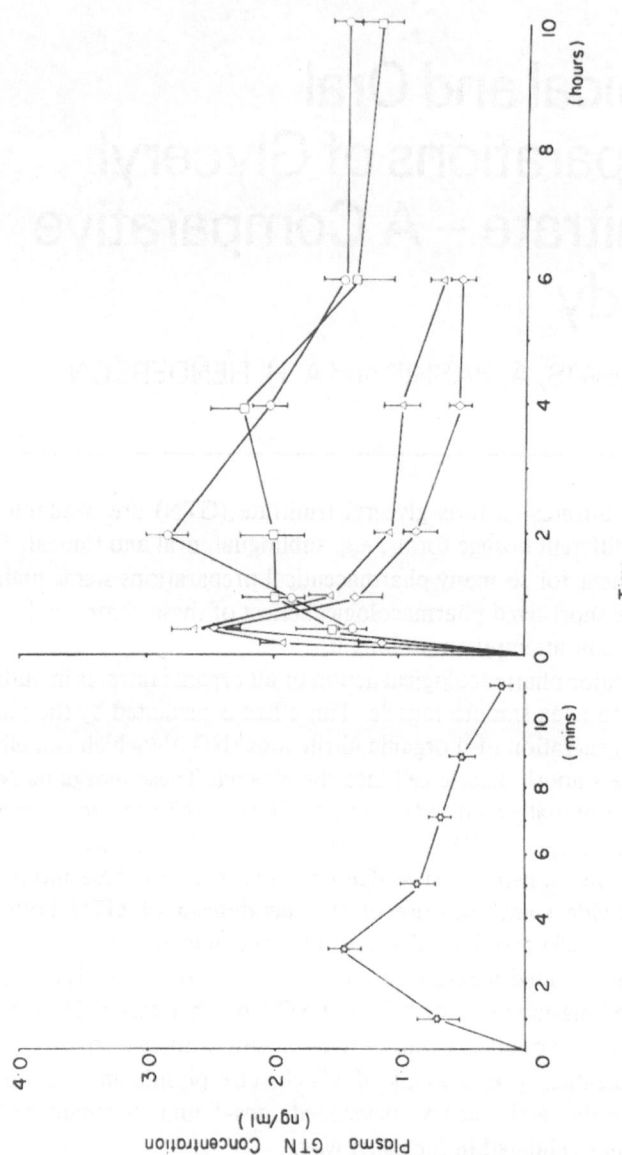

Figure 1 Mean (± SEM) plasma GTN levels following administration of sublingual GTN (☆); Nitrocontin (○); Sustac (□); GTN cream (△); and GTN ointment (◇)

In each case the preparation was given at 10.00h, after an overnight fast. Ingestion of canned foods, which are a potent source of NO_2^-, was avoided for > 3 days before the study. Venous blood samples were taken and simple haemodynamic measurements of heart rate and blood pressure made in the supine position.

Sublingual GTN (0.5mg) was administered by placing a tablet under the tongue for 5min. Two slow-release GTN preparations, Nitrocontin and Sustac (each containing 6.4mg GTN) were given orally. Doses of GTN cream and GTN ointment (containing 23mg and 35mg GTN respectively) were administered by applying 2.5in, from a standard dispensing tube to the anterior chest wall, spreading to cover an area of 36in^2 and covered with a polythene sheet for 6h.

Figure 1 shows the blood levels of GTN. After sublingual GTN, peak levels of 1.4ng/ml were reached in about 3min. The peak levels with the two topical preparations and the two slow-release oral preparations were approximately similar at about 2.5–2.8ng/ml, almost double the level after sublingual GTN. Note also that peak levels were reached earlier after the topical preparations than after the slow-release preparations.

Comparison of the area under the curves (AUC) of the two oral and two topical preparations, which provides information on the bio-availability of the preparations (Table 1) shows no significant differences between the two oral forms but the cream had a

Table 1   Mean ($\pm$ SEM) of the areas under the curves (AUCs) of the two oral and two topical GTN preparations $(ng\,ml^{-1}h^{-1})$

Nitrocontin	18.0 ± 1.1
Sustac	16.5 ± 2.1
Ointment	5.2 ± 0.01
Cream	7.1 ± 1.6*

* $p < 0.05$ for comparison of cream and ointment

significantly greater AUC than the ointment, despite containing a lower content of GTN. This indicates a greater bioavailability of GTN from the cream than from the ointment, probably related to the lower solubility of GTN in a water-based cream than the oil-based ointment.

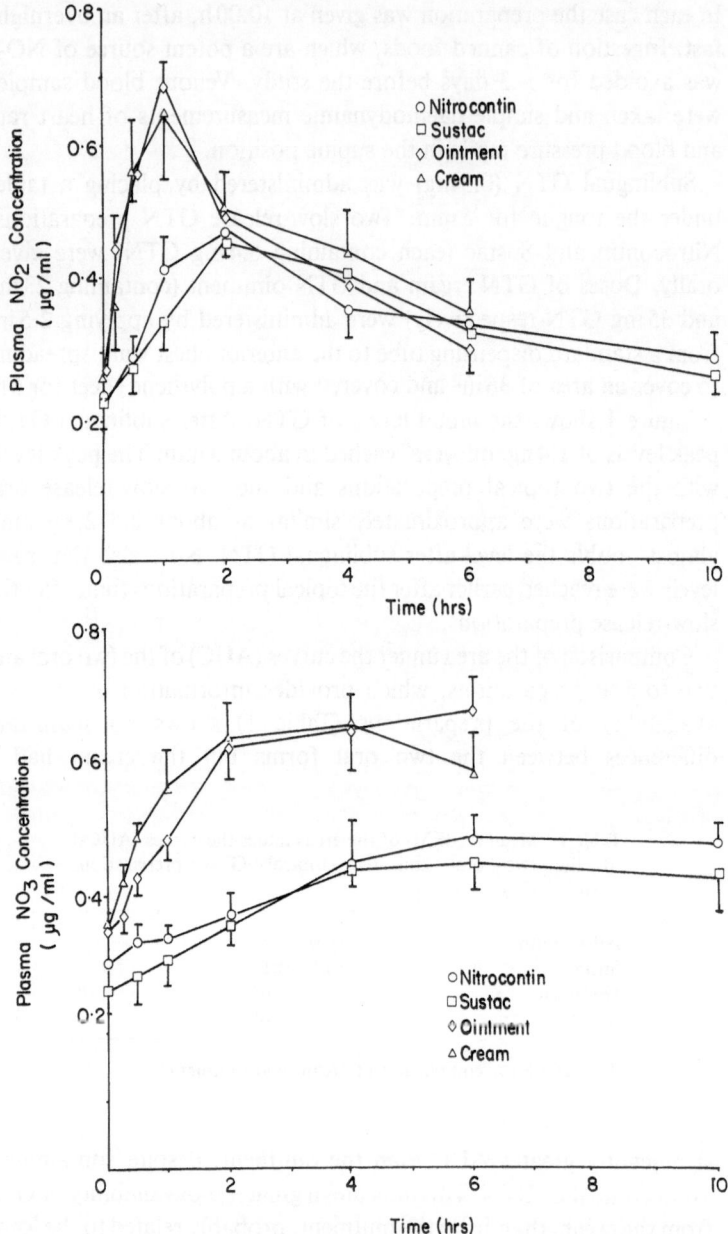

Figure 2   Mean (± SEM) plasma levels of NO_3^- and NO_2^- following administration of Nitrocontin, Sustac, GTN cream and ointment

Figure 2 shows the findings with NO_3^- and NO_2^-. No increase in these was detected after sublingual GTN. Following the topical preparations a level of about $0.7\,\mu g/ml$ of both NO_3^- and NO_2^- was reached and after the slow-release preparations about $0.5\,\mu g/ml$ of both ions. The levels of NO_3^- and NO_2^- reached after the topical preparations were significantly greater than after the oral preparations. This is of obvious interest since it suggests that degradation of the GTN is greater during absorption through the skin than during absorption through the gut.

The question of obvious importance is whether these NO_3^- and NO_2^- ions generated from the intracellular metabolism of GTN exert a pharmacological effect. Very little data is available comparing the vasodilator properties of different organic and inorganic nitrates. What data is available in animals[2] suggests that NO_3^- has little or no pharmacological action. Inorganic NO_2^-, however, has about one-fourtieth to one-fiftieth the vasodilator action of GTN. Because the plasma levels of NO_2^-, however, are about 200 times that of GTN itself we can estimate that the vasodilator effect of NO_2^- is four to five times that of the GTN. Further work to validate these findings is obviously needed, but it emphasizes the need to measure the levels of all relevant metabolites in pharmacokinetic studies of these rather complicated drugs.

Figure 3 shows the heart rate and systolic and diastolic blood pressure responses after the five preparations. Both the blood pressure and heart rate responses were significantly greater following sublingual GTN than either of the oral preparations when measured at the time of the respective peak GTN plasma levels, despite the much lower plasma GTN levels after sublingual GTN. In other words we get a greater haemodynamic response with a lower GTN level and no detectable rise in NO_2^-. There is, however, a considerable difference in the duration of exposure to the GTN. Peak levels and haemodynamic response was at 3 min after sublingual GTN compared with $\frac{1}{2}$–2h after the other preparations. This suggests that tolerance is developing extremely rapidly over this time.

Comparison of the haemodynamic changes at the time of peak plasma GTN after the slow-release and topical preparations shows that although the differences did not reach statistical significance, the changes after the topical preparations were greater than after the slow-release preparations despite similar peak plasma GTN levels.

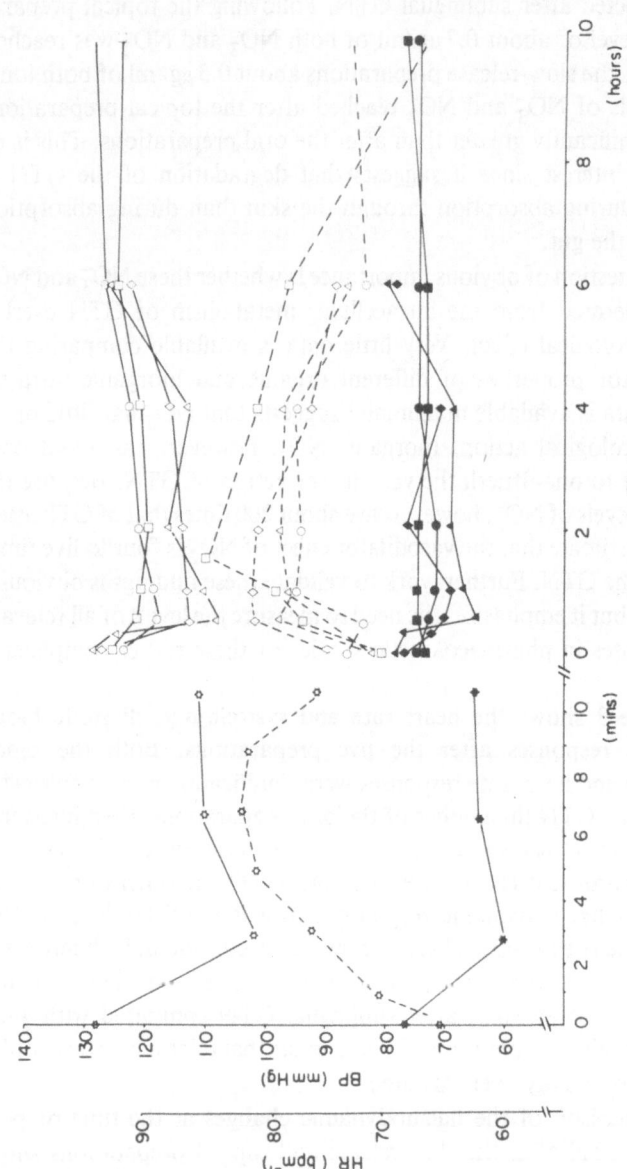

Figure 3   Mean HR (broken lines), systolic BP (open symbols, solid lines) and diastolic BP (closed symbols, solid lines) after sublingual GTN (☆); Nitrocontin (○); Sustac (□); GTN cream (△); and ointment (◇)

The differences here could also be explained by differences in the times of peak exposure to GTN, i.e. about $\frac{1}{2}$ h after topical administration and about 2 h after oral administration. There is also the complicating effect of the NO_2^- levels, however, which were slightly greater after the topical preparations and could therefore account for this difference.

In summary we have shown that oral and topical administration of GTN produced higher and more sustained plasma levels than after sublingual administration, the higher levels being tolerated perhaps because of the rapid development of tolerance. Secondly, there is little difference in the oral preparations studied but the cream showed a higher bioavailability than the ointment despite containing a smaller amount of GTN. Thirdly, plasma NO_3^- and NO_2^- levels were higher after the topical preparations than after the oral preparations despite similar peak GTN levels, implying metabolism of GTN during passage through the skin. Finally, when measured at the time of peak GTN levels, the haemodynamic changes of the oral and topical preparations were much smaller than after sublingual GTN, indicating the very rapid development of tolerance over less than 1 h.

Acknowledgement

We would like to thank Napp Laboratories Ltd., who provided the financial support for the studies.

References

1. Needleman, P. and Hunter, F. E. (1965). The transformation of glyceryl trinitrate and other nitrates by glutathione organic nitrate reductase. *Mol. Pharmacol.*, **9**, 77
2. Needleman, P., Blehm, D. J. and Rotskoff, K. S. (1969). Relationship between glutathione-dependent denitration and the vasodilator effectiveness of organic nitrates. *J. Pharmacol. Exp. Ther.*, **165**, 286
3. Needleman, P. (1976). Organic nitrate metabolism. *Ann. Rev. Pharmacol. Toxicol.*, **16**, 81

11
The Influence of Formulation on Percutaneous Absorption

I. W. KELLAWAY

The principal objectives of the formulator of topical medicinal products are to design a dosage form which is both chemically and physically stable and is cosmetically acceptable. In addition, there is the need to ensure that the vehicle provides optimal delivery of the drug to the target tissues. Effective therapy will only be achieved if the various interactions and actions resulting post-application of the dosage form to the skin surface occur in a controlled manner. Drug release, penetration and target activity are dependent on the inter-actions occurring between drug, vehicle and skin. Vehicle–drug inter-actions will determine the drug release profile, whilst vehicle–skin interactions can modulate the penetration phase.

DRUG VEHICLE EFFECTS

Two interdependent diffusional processes occur in the transdermal delivery of drugs. The first is the release of drug from the vehicle; the second the penetration of the skin barrier. The mechanisms associated with the release phase will be different for drugs formu-lated as a solution or as a dispersion, i.e. suspension. If formulated as a solution, drug release rate is represented by the equation

$$dQ/dt = C_0(D/\pi t)^{0.5} \quad \text{for } Q < 30\% \tag{1}$$

and for a suspension

$$dQ/dt = 1/2 \left[\frac{D(2C_0 - C_v)C_v}{t} \right]^{0.5}$$

(2)

which simplifies when $C_0 >> C_v t$

$$dQ/dt = \left(\frac{C_0 C_v D}{2t} \right)^{0.5}$$

(3)

where dQ/dt = rate of drug released to the skin surface per unit area;

C_0 = initial drug concentration in the vehicle (suspended and dissolved);

C_v = solubility of the drug in the vehicle;

D = diffusivity of the drug in the vehicle;

and t = time at which the amount of drug released is determined.

From these equations it is evident that release rate can be controlled by manipulation of C_0 and D for solution formulations and C_0, C_v and D for suspensions. The diffusivity is inversely proportional to the viscosity of the surrounding media or microenvironment of the diffusing species. However, with structural phases such as those encountered in many topical vehicles, bulk viscosity measurements have little value in the evaluation of resistance to the movement of penetrant molecules. If the penetrant molecules contain groups capable of hydrogen bonding, greatly reduced diffusivity may result compared with molecules of similar molecular volume. Suspensions offer the possibility of ensuring that the rate-limiting step in the overall transport process is that of drug release. Examination of equations (1)–(3) indicates that for a given drug concentration, release will be faster from a vehicle in which the drug is completely soluble. Doubling the concentration of drug in a suspension formulation results in a release rate increase of approximately 40%.

SKIN PENETRATION

Because vehicle release and skin penetration are interrelated diffusional processes, it is pertinent to examine the factors influencing the flux of drug (J) across the skin barrier, which for these purposes can be treated as a simple membrane.

$$J = \frac{K_m D_m \Delta C_s}{h} \qquad (4)$$

where K_m = partition coefficient between the membrane and the applied vehicle;

$\quad\quad D_m$ = diffusivity of drug in the membrane;

$\quad\quad h$ = membrane thickness;

and ΔC_s = concentration difference of drug across the membrane.

If the skin is regarded as a perfect sink, then equation (4) may be simplified to give

$$J = \frac{K_m D_m C_v}{h} \qquad (5)$$

To enhance penetration, vehicle development has been directed along two principal routes. Firstly, agents can be included in the vehicle that reversibly affect the barrier function of the epidermis, so as to promote penetration of the therapeutic compound. These agents primarily serve to increase D_m by various mechanisms. Secondly, the physical characteristics of the vehicle can be altered, thus affecting the diffusion of the drug from the vehicle into the skin. In this case flux is being increased by manipulation of K_m and C_v.

PARTITION COEFFICIENT (K_m) AND SOLUBILITY (C_v)

Although partition coefficients of penetrants have often been determined in various two-phase systems, such determinations are of limited value compared with partitioning studies using samples of stratum corneum and the vehicle being developed. K_m is a measure of the relative affinity of the penetrant for the stratum corneum and the vehicle. Although frequently expressed as the ratio of concentrations in the respective phases, the true partition coefficient is defined as the ratio of the thermodynamic activities. The use of activity rather than concentration is particularly important where there is self-association of the penetrant or complexation of the penetrant with vehicle components. For a given concentration of drug in certain vehicles, the activity may vary by as much as 1000-fold from one vehicle to the next[1]. Penetrants held 'firmly' by the vehicle exhibit low activity coefficients and consequently, release rates are slow. Conversely, penetrants 'loosely' held within the vehicle exhibit high activity coefficients and thus the release rates are faster. The influence of vehicle on K_m can be demonstrated by reference to studies by Scheuplein[2], who examined the permeability of ethanol and heptanol from single-component vehicles. The polar ethanol was shown to penetrate better from hydrophobic oils than water, whereas the reverse was true for the less polar heptanol. Thus, the more polar solute tends to remain in the most polar vehicle and not be transferred to the skin; transference did, however, occur from oily vehicles.

The solubility of a drug within a vehicle is often enhanced by the use of cosolvents, for example propylene glycol will increase steroid solubility in aqueous vehicles. However, such solubility increases usually result in reduced partition coefficients[3]. Maximum release rates are achieved from vehicles containing the minimum amount of propylene glycol required for drug solubility. The product $K_m.C_v$ is often a more powerful index of drug availability than either parameter alone.

The efficiency of vehicles in aiding penetration can often be related to their effect on hydration of the stratum corneum or the activity of water within the stratum corneum which influences the stratum corneum–vehicle partition coefficient. Thus any vehicle inducing hydration through sweat accumulation at the vehicle – skin interface has the potential for enhancing penetration[4]. Greases and oils are amongst the most occlusive vehicles, although the use of occlusive bandages or polymer films is often more effective.

EMULSIONS

The literature on the influence of emulsions on skin penetration is confusing and often contradictory. The observed effects may result from penetrant partitioning between the emulsion phases, the participation of the surfactants in the transport process or a combination of such processes. The role of preservatives in such formulations, and the possibility of cracking or phase inversion on application to the skin surface, severely limits our understanding of this complex system.

When the epidermis is treated with surfactants its permeability to water alters. The observed irritant effect of anionic surfactants suggests that such compounds are capable of penetration. Although penetration is generally poor, the order of effectiveness is anionics >cationics>non-ionics[5]. A carbon chain length of 12 results in maximum penetration amongst anionics and also exerts the greatest influence on other penetrants[6,7]. Long-chain sulphonated fatty acids begin to penetrate the dermis only after saturation of the epidermis. Anionics bind strongly to skin proteins causing a reversible denaturation manifested as an uncoiling of the filaments, causing expansion of the tissues[8]. The conformational changes in the protein brought about by anionic–surfactant binding, may result in the polar groups being forced into the interior of the helices. This would explain the enhanced skin penetration of water and hydrophilic compounds in the presence of anionic surfactants. The hydrophilic–lipophilic balance (HLB) has been investigated as an explanation of non-ionic surfactant effects[9] on the flux of oestradiol and progesterone from Tween 60/Span 60 stabilized oil-in-water emulsions applied to the skin. Oestradiol flux was inversely related to the HLB whilst progesterone flux was independent of HLB. The latter was explained by the high oil/water (low stratum corneum/oil) partition coefficients observed for progesterone, suggesting that progesterone remains strongly associated with the dispersed oil phase.

COLLOIDAL DRUG CARRIERS

Recently multilamellar liposomes containing triamcinolone acetonide formulated as a lotion[10] were shown in rabbits to increase the levels of steroid in the epidermis and dermis compared with control (non-liposomal) formulations. The transport of intact vehicles across the skin is unlikely, yet drug disposition was shown to be significantly different from control preparations. However, the washing of the skin surface with ethanol prior to sacrifice, which would destroy the liposome integrity and yield local, high drug activity at the skin surface, may in part explain the reported drug loading of the epidermis and dermis. Other potential lipophilic colloidal delivery systems include microemulsions.

SUMMARY

The often conflicting reports on the relative merits of vehicles in influencing skin penetration arise from the diversity of the methodologies employed. Different methods have been used to estimate skin penetration in various *in vitro* systems or in a variety of animal models. Perhaps of greater significance is a failure to appreciate the structure and interactions occurring within multi-component vehicles which can lead to dramatic changes in the thermodynamic activities of the formulated penetrant.

References

1. Higuchi, T. (1960). Physical chemical analysis of percutaneous absorption process from creams and ointments. *J. Soc. Cosmet. Chem.,* **11,** 85–97
2. Scheuplein, R. J. (1965). Mechanism of percutaneous absorption. 1. Routes of penetration and influence of solubility. *J. Invest. Dermatol.,* **45,** 334–346
3. Katz, M. and Poulsen, B. J. (1972). Corticoid, vehicle and skin interaction in percutaneous absorption. *J. Soc. Cosmet. Chem.,* **23,** 565–590
4. Shelmire, J. B. (1960). Factors determining the skin–drug–vehicle relationship. *Arch. Dermatol.,* **82,** 24–31
5. Bettley, F. R. (1965). Influence of detergents and surfactants on epidermal permeability. *Br. J. Dermatol.,* **77,** 98–100
6. Bettley, F. R. (1961). Influence of soap on the permeability of the epidermis. *Br. J. Dermatol.,* **73,** 448–454
7. Bettley, F. R. (1963). Irritant effect of soap in relation to epidermal permeability. *Br. J. Dermatol.,* **75,** 113–116
8. Scheuplein, R. J. and Ross, L. (1970). Effects of surfactants and solvents on the permeability of epidermis. *J. Soc. Cosmet. Chem.,* **21,** 853–873
9. Wepierre, J. and Marty, J. P. (1977). Rôle des excipients et des agents tensio-actifs dans l'absorption percutanée des substances chimiques. *Gattefossé Report,* pp. 53–59
10. Mezei, M. and Gulasekharam, V. (1980). Liposomes – a selective drug delivery system for the topical route of administration. *Life Sci.,* **26,** 1473–1477

12
Pharmacological and Physical Measurement of Drug Penetration into Skin

M. I. FOREMAN

The problem being addressed here may be stated as: 'given a molecule with potential local activity in skin, how may the molecule be modified so as to maximize both its intrinsic pharmacological effect and its skin penetration ability?'

The ideal empirical approach would be to synthesize a series of analogues of a particular drug, and then compare their potencies in patients suffering from the specific disease of interest. In general, this approach is not possible, since toxicity testing etc. before human use may be contemplated would be prohibitively expensive. Even if it were possible, however, very large numbers of patients would almost certainly be required to provide the necessary discriminatory power. One exception is the human vasoconstrictor (HVC) test for corticosteroids. Here, the application of minute amounts of corticosteroids to skin induces a blanching response, the intensity of which has long been considered to correlate with local anti-inflammatory potency in humans. This has therefore been the basis of methodology employed by various groups to obtain potency comparisons between corticosteroids, based on their combined potency and penetrative power. In some cases a separation of the two effects is possible. The steroid rimexolone (11β-hydroxy-16α, 17α-21-trimethyl-pregna-1,4-diene-3,20-dione) induces an HVC response having an appreciably faster onset than, for example, beta-methasone valerate (Figure 1), which implies a more rapid penetrative ability for this compound[1]. Since the peak activity therefore occurs at

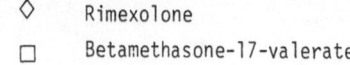

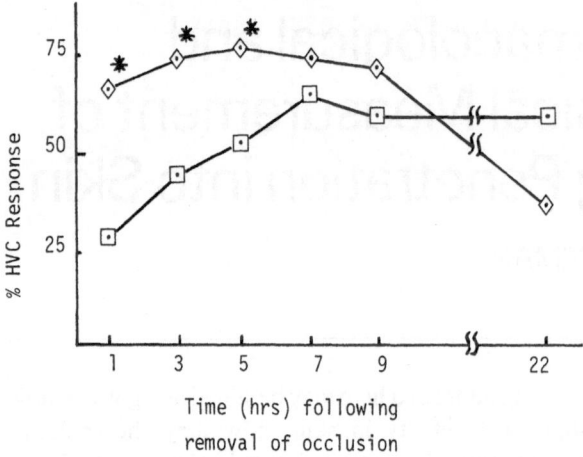

Time (hrs) following
removal of occlusion

* Significantly different P ⩽ 0.05

Figure 1 HVC response induced by rimexolone and betamethasone-17-valerate as a function of time following 3-h application under plastic occlusion

an earlier time, comparisons of inherent clinical activity require a separate study with the timing of the drug administration modified to allow the peak responses to occur simultaneously, and direct comparisons to be made. Under such circumstances, the separate contributions of penetration and intrinsic activity have therefore, in effect, been compared, making the reasonable assumption that the response at the receptor level is much faster than the penetration process.

A second approach uses animal studies, where much more complex measurements are possible. Drug tissue distribution, blood levels and excretion rates may all be monitored to assess the efficacy of penetration of topically applied material. Such studies can also, of course, be combined with measurement of a relevant pharmacological response. In this approach, however, the greater sophistication of the measurement must be offset against the very real problems of the possible lack of relevance of such animal models to the human situation, and this may be especially true when considering minor modifications on a basic drug molecule rather than gross differences between drugs.

So far as the two former approaches are concerned, most practical applications are empirical, going no further than simply comparing one drug, or drug/vehicle combination, with another. This is perfectly acceptable, and certainly provides a powerful tool for drug development. For the longer term, however, fundamental information is necessary to allow a more rational basis for the design of drugs and vehicles for topical use. In this respect, some form of *in vitro* model system employing excised human skin has decided advantages. The process of vehicle application, drug release from the vehicle, interactions at the skin/vehicle interface, and drug migration through the skin may be modelled under more controlled circumstances.

Whether *in vivo* or *in vitro* methods are employed, however, where studies of drug diffusion in skin are concerned, a general problem which arises is that the basic second-order differential equations which describe the diffusion process are only solvable for a limited number of specific boundary conditions. One solution, due originally to Daynes[2], reduces to a rather simple mathematical equation under one specific set of circumstances, which form the basis for an elegantly simple experimental design[3]. This has, therefore, been employed in most skin penetration studies to date (see, for example, Scheuplein *et al.*[4]). Unfortunately, this method requires that the skin sample is in constant contact with water, on both sides, throughout the experiment. This inevitably produces a situation where the sample becomes saturated with water, and since it is well known that skin hydration has marked effects on drug diffusion, the rather unphysiologically high levels of tissue hydration achieved in these experiments bring into question the relevance of much of this work. In general, the boundary conditions for which the basic equations are solvable pay no regard to the needs of the experimenter, and this has restricted severely the study of drug diffusion in skin up to the present time.

There is an alternative approach which has wide generality, which will undoubtedly prove useful in other circumstances, and which frees the experimenter from the restrictions of the traditional analytical mathematical approach. Drug diffusion is in fact a process of simple random molecular motion, and, in one sense, therefore, analytical mathematical approaches are 'artificial'. Modern computers now being cheap to buy and to run, it becomes a simple matter to simulate diffusion behaviour as a process of random molecular motion under any set of boundary conditions. Specifically: normal 'physiological' skin is bounded on the lower side by an effectively infinite sink (the vascular system), and on the other it is open to the air. Drug administration is usually as a finite dose in a thin film to the upper surface, which may or may not then be occluded. This situation is not amenable to analytical solution, but can easily be simulated.

The computer predicted curve which results from such a simulation[5] is perfectly general. All experimental curves under these conditions will have the same general shape, and can be adjusted, by applying a scaling factor to the *x*-axis of the experimental curve, to an

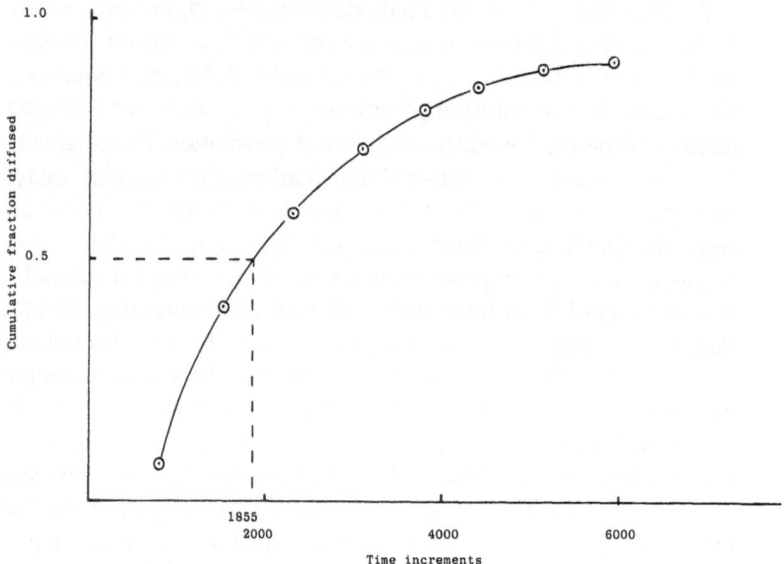

Figure 2 Simulated diffusion curve for material applied to a plane membrane of thickness L, penetrating with diffusion constant D into an infinite sink.

Each time increment = real time $\times S_t$,

where $S_t = \dfrac{(L/50)^2}{2D}$

$T_{\frac{1}{2}}^{D}$ = time for one half of the diffusant to penetrate the membrane = $1855 \times S_t$ (from the simulation) = $0.371 \, L^2/D$

identical shape to that predicted by the computer (in practice this means 'best least-squares fit' between the curves). The scaling factor provides an estimate of the function L^2/D where L is the skin thickness. D may then be obtained from a knowledge of L.

A number of advantages are immediately apparent using this method. For example, since a finite dose has been applied, it is possible to characterize the diffusion of a specific drug in terms of the time taken for one-half of the applied dose to penetrate ($T_{\frac{1}{2}}^D$) (Figure 2)[6]. This is a much more easily assimilated concept, in some respects, than a diffusion constant. It represents the nett barrier of the skin to a specific drug, and is easily calculated from the equation $T_{\frac{1}{2}}^D = 0.371 L^2/D$, which means that it is a more accurately derived parameter than D, since a knowledge of L is not required.

In conclusion, it must be said that both the empirical and more fundamental approaches described above are of value. Rational development of drugs for transdermal administration demands, however, a basis of fundamental understanding of the broader aspects of the nature of skin as a diffusion barrier, along with a detailed knowledge of specific aspects of the problem which seem of immediate relevance. Computer simulation of diffusion processes in skin seems likely to offer considerable advantages in this respect, and it is hoped that advances will be made in what remains at present the least well understood method of drug delivery.

References

1. Clanachan, I., Devitt, H. G., Foreman, M. I. and Kelly, I. P. (1980). The human vasoconstrictor assay for topical steroids. *J. Pharmacol. Meth.*, **4**, 209–220
2. Daynes, H. (1920). The process of diffusion through a rubber membrane. *Proc. Roy. Soc.*, **A97**, 286
3. Barrer, R. M. (1951). *Diffusion in and through Solids*, 1st Edn., p. 18. (Cambridge: Cambridge University Press)
4. Scheuplein, R. J., Blank, I. H., Brauner, G. J. and MacFarlane, D. J. (1969). Percutaneous absorption of steroids. *J. Invest. Dermatol.*, **52**, 63–70
5. Foreman, M. I., Kelly, I. and Lukowiecki, G. A. (1977). A method for the measurement of diffusion constants suitable for studies of non-occluded skin. *J. Pharm. Pharmacol.*, **29**, 108
6. Foreman, M. I., Clanachan, I. and Kelly, I. P. (1983). Diffusion barriers in skin – a new method of comparison. *Br. J. Dermatol.*, **108**, 549–553

Index